Th

Richard Mackarness MB, BS, DPM, was educated at Lancing and qualified at the Westminster Hospital School of Medicine. After service in the RAMC, he joined an educational filmstrip company where he designed the pictures and wrote the teaching notes for filmstrips on health subjects. There followed a period as a hospital registrar after which he worked for two years as medical adviser to a pharmaceutical company before setting up in general practice under the NHS. In 1965 he moved to Park Prewett Hospital, Basingstoke, as a psychiatric registrar, and obtained the Diploma in Psychological Medicine (DPM). In 1967 he was appointed to the permanent staff as Assistant Psychiatrist.

Recent work has included research on clinical ecology (the role of the non-living environment, foods and chemicals particularly, in the development of obesity and mental illness). Dr Mackarness now runs an obesity/food allergy clinic at Basingstoke District Hospital. It is the first of its kind in Britain.

Dr Mackarness started to write on medical matters in 1956 when he became Medical Correspondent of the *News Chronicle*.

Eat Fat and Grow Slim

Richard Mackarness
MB, BS, DPM

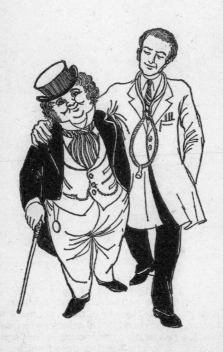

Fontana/Collins

First published by the Harvill Press 1958
First issued in Fontana Paperbacks 1961

This new, revised, and extended edition
first published 1975

Illustrations by Zelma Mackenzie
Diagrams by William Jones
Copyright © Richard Mackarness 1958, 1975

Made and printed in Great Britain by
William Collins Sons and Co Ltd, Glasgow

To the Memory of Sir Robert McCarrison
whose pioneering work on nutrition and
health has been an inspiration to me

Contents

Acknowledgements

I wish to thank all those people without whose help and encouragement I could never have completed this revised version of my book. First, the medical and nursing staff of the Basingstoke District Hospital at Park Prewett who have referred fat patients to me and have helped me to slim them, using methods described in this book. Likewise the general practitioners of North Hampshire who have entrusted some of their very fat patients to me. I particularly want to thank Mrs Slade, the Dietician, and Mr Wadley, the Catering Officer, who have co-operated so well with me in providing patients with their diets; Sister Hawkins and the staff of Upton Ward for their enthusiastic application of the High-Fibre diet to the old ladies on that ward; Dr Gaston Pawan of the Middlesex Hospital who has kept me up to date with his research and that of the late Professor Alan Kekwick on the Fat Mobilizing Hormone; Eliza Kendall of *Vogue* magazine who read and sub-edited the manuscript, and Leslie Kenton of *Harpers and Queen* who provided the basis for the Wholefood Diet in Appendix C; my fellow-members of the McCarrison Society who have taught me so much.

The late Dr Vilhjalmur Stefansson, Arctic explorer and anthropologist, whose book, *The Fat of the Land*, has given me more information than any other, besides being a pleasure to read (extracts from *The Fat of the Land*, 1956, are included by kind permission of the Macmillan Company of New York); Dr Robert Kemp and *Medical News Magazine* for permission to quote from his speech at their symposium on obesity; my good friend Dr Wolfgang Lutz of Salzburg and his publisher Selecta-Verlag; Dr Ildar Idris, for permission to quote from his book, *Leben ohne Brot* (Life without Bread); Dr Barbara Latto and *World Medicine* whose Science Editor quoted her McCarrison-type diet in the 8 September 1971 issue of that magazine; Dr K. W. Heaton and the publishers of *The Lancet* for permission to quote his letter on food fibre and obesity; Surgeon Captain Cleave, Dr Campbell and Professor N. S. Painter and their publishers, John Wright & Sons of Bristol, for permission to quote from their book *Diabetes, Coronary Thrombosis and the Saccharine Disease*; Professor J. N. Morris and *The Lancet* for permission to quote his letter about the epidemiology of heart attacks; Professor Jean Mayer of Harvard for permission to quote from his speech on genetic factors in obesity; Mrs Doris Grant for permission to quote her recipe for the Grant Loaf.

I wish to thank all those readers of the earlier version of *Eat Fat and Grow Slim* who wrote to tell me that they had managed to slim by this method, and the doctors in America who I visited after the book was published over there and who encouraged me by telling me that I was on the right lines: Dr Stefansson, Dr Alfred Pennington, Dr Ray Lawson, Dr George Thorpe, Dr Don Mitchell and Dr Ted Randolph. My secretary, Marjorie Hurst for all her help, and my wife and son for their tolerance of my neglect of the garden and the carpentry at home while I was doing this revision.

Finally, Zelma MacKenzie, who has redrawn the chapter headpieces and done some new ones and Peter Grose of Curtis Brown who could not be a better agent.

R.M. 1974

Preface

It is now more than sixteen years since I wrote *Eat Fat and Grow Slim*. Since then a lot of work has been done on obesity, but the basic argument still remains unresolved, with the two sides shouting as loudly as ever: one claiming that it is all a matter of over-eating and gluttony, the other (to which I belong) that it is a little-understood metabolic difference between fat and thin people.

The gluttony school believes in the efficacy of calorie counting and has considerable commercial backing from the food and slimming-aid industry. The metabolic-defect school has now a lot more evidence to back up its arguments, not only from research physiologists, but from anthropologists and clinicians who have studied fat and thin people in action.

As the readers of the original edition of *Eat Fat and Grow Slim* will know, it is to this latter school that I belong. My central arguments concerning food and its relation to health remain in essence as before. But in this new edition I have presented fresh evidence and taken into account much of the work in this field done by others since the first edition was published. This has involved the writing of three new chapters and the rewriting of the others.

There are many different ways of slimming, from fasting to surgical operations, and in Chapter 7 I have given an account of these various methods. But however you go about losing weight, the final problem is always the same: how do you avoid putting it back on again? I think I have the answer to this. In fact I had it in the earlier version of the book. But now two things have changed concerning our food. First, it has become much more expensive, especially meat and fish. Secondly it has become much more adulterated and refined in order to fit it for the supermarket style of distribution, which was only just beginning when I wrote the earlier version of this book.

A third factor which must now be considered is the appalling rise in the number of deaths from coronary thrombosis and strokes (now over 500,000 per year in the United States alone!), and the linking by some doctors of this epidemic of cardio-vascular disease which may or may not be associated with overweight, with the consumption of animal fats, particularly cholesterol.

I am convinced that the animal fat and cholesterol scare is a red herring in the search for the cause or causes of coronary thrombosis, and in Chapter 4 I give my reasons for saying this. Here I would like to say that it is inconceivable that a food (fat meat) which has been man's staple diet for nine-tenths of his time as a human, should suddenly become the cause of a disease which was unknown before the turn of the century. And even more inconceivable is the idea that choles-terol is to blame, since this fatty substance is an essential part of the body's economy. The fact that a raised level of cholesterol is found in the blood of some (but not all) people who die of coronary thrombosis does *not* prove that the cholesterol caused the heart attack. One of the commonest flaws in so-called scientific arguments today is to assume that because one thing follows another, the first caused the second. You might just as well say that because more black people than white people have malaria, malaria is caused by having a coloured skin.

It is more likely that obesity *and* coronary thrombosis have a common cause in what we are doing to our diet in Western countries, and it is this aspect of the matter which I have developed in this new edition of my book.

Too few people realize that in the last fifty to seventy years, the food manufacturing industry in Western countries has been allowed, with Government acquiescence, to carry out a nutri-tional experiment of extreme foolhardiness: I refer to the refining and concentration of carbohydrate to make white flour and sugar and the addition of thousands of synthetic chemicals to foods of all kinds, at every stage from the farm to the supermarket. Mankind has evolved slowly and painfully on a diet based first on a gatherer-type, monkey diet of leaves, fruit and seeds, and secondly on free-running fat meat hunted on the wide savannah after the rain forests shrank some two to three million years ago.

Only in the last few seconds of man's evolutionary day has he been fed a diet based on cereal grains – 6000 to 10,000 years at most – and only for a fraction of a second has he had to eat synthetic chemicals in the form of pesticides put into the ground and sprayed on crops, flour 'improvers', artificial colourings, anti-staling agents, emulsifying compounds, synthetic flavours and the whole terrifying array of potentially harmful new substances now being added to our food to improve its appearance, flavour, shelf-life and profitability.

It is no coincidence that the onset and progress of the three-fold epidemic of obesity, heart disease and behaviour disorders which now afflicts Western society should exactly parallel the refining, concentration and chemical sophistication of diet. The evidence for a causal relationship is overwhelming, as this new edition of my book will show, calling on evidence from history, anthropology and medical research. Time is running out. Unless we force the Government to reverse its food policies and go back to unadulterated whole food – including the essential fats on which our brains and nerves evolved – obesity will cease to be a major problem because we will go the way of the dinosaurs and the dodo and become extinct.

BIBLIOGRAPHY AND REFERENCES

As this book has been written primarily for non-medical people, the text has not been cluttered up with references and footnotes. For doctors and others who wish to check my sources, a note of books consulted and references to journal articles is given at the end of each chapter.

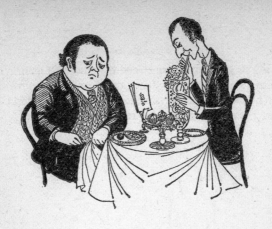

I

What Makes a Fat Person Fat?

People can be divided into two groups according to how they deal with the excess when they eat more than they need for their daily expenditure of energy.

In 1950, at the Royal Society of Medicine in London, Professor Sir Charles Dodds, who was in charge of the Courtauld Institute of Biochemistry at the Middlesex Hospital, described an experiment he had carried out. He took people whose weights had been constant for many years and persuaded them to eat double or treble their normal amount of food. They did not put on weight. He showed that this was not due to a failure to digest or assimilate the extra food and suggested that they responded to over-eating by increasing their metabolic rate (rate of food using) and thus burned up the extra calories.

He then over-fed people whose weights had not remained constant in the past and found that they showed no increase in metabolism but became fat.

So two people of the same size, doing the same work and eating the same food will react differently when they over-eat.

One will stay the same weight and the other will gain.

Since Sir Charles Dodds carried out his experiment, research doctors and physiologists all over the world have repeated it and confirmed his results.

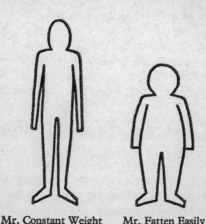

Mr. Constant Weight   Mr. Fatten Easily

Any intelligent person knows that this is a true difference between two basic sorts of people, yet the fact has not been taken into account or explained by any of the experts who write popular books and articles about slimming.

They write as though fat people and thin people deal with food in the same way. Here is the medical correspondent of *The Times* on the subject: 'It is no use saying as so many women do: "But I eat practically nothing." The only answer to this is: "No matter how little you imagine you eat, if you wish to lose weight you must eat less." Your reserves of fat are then called on to provide the necessary energy – and you lose weight.'

The doctor who wrote these rather heartless words may fairly be taken as representative of medical opinion today.

He is applying the teachings of William Wadd, Surgeon-Extraordinary to the Prince Regent, who in 1829 attributed obesity to 'an over-indulgence at the table' and gave, as the first principle of treatment, 'taking food that has little nutrition in it'.

Fat people can certainly lose weight by this method but what do they feel like while they are doing it? Absolutely terrible.

Ask any fat person who has tried it. Many of these unfortunate people really do eat less than people of normal proportions *and still they put on weight,* and when they go on a strict low-calorie diet which does get weight off, they feel tired and irritable because they are subjecting themselves to starvation. Worse still, when they have reduced and feel they can eat a little more, up shoots their weight again in no time, on quite a moderate food intake.

It is all most discouraging. 'Surely there must be some better way of going about it,' they say. This book explains that there is. Today a lot more is known about how fat people get fat and why. Many of the facts have been known for years, but because they have not fitted in with current theories on obesity, they have been ignored.

In the last ten years, however, atomic research has given the physiologist enormous help in unravelling the biochemical reactions which go on in the body.

Radio-active isotopes have been used to 'tag' chemical substances so that their progress through the body could be followed, in the same way as birds are tagged in order to establish the paths of their migration.

By this means, details of the metabolism of fats and carbohydrates, previously shrouded in mystery, have been clarified and with the new information so gained old experimental findings have been given new interpretations and the jigsaw of seemingly contradictory facts about obesity has clicked into a recognizable picture.

The first thing to realize is that it is carbohydrate (starch and sugar) and *carbohydrate only* which fattens fat people.

When Mr Constant-Weight has too much starch and sugar to eat, he automatically stokes up his body fires, increasing his metabolism, so the excess calories are consumed. Nothing is left over for laying down as fat, and his weight remains unchanged.

The physiological mechanisms which enable him to do this are remarkably precise and it is an amazing fact that Constant-Weights like Abraham Lincoln, Bertrand Russell, Lord Home and actor James Stewart could and can eat as they wish, varying their intake from day to day without conscious reference to the amount of physical exercise they take, and yet remain the same weight to within a pound or two, all their lives.

When a Fatten-Easily like Hubert Humphrey, Cyril Smith, MP, or Chairman Mao eats too much bread, sugar or cake, the picture is different: there is evidence that he is less active anyway than his lean brothers and that his metabolic fires burn at a lower rate most of the time. Even his basic calorie ration, if taken as carbohydrate, tends to go to fat rather than use, and if he takes an excess of starch and sugar, this depresses his metabolism further and weight is gained easily. Why does he fail to burn up the excess? The answer is the real reason for his obesity: BECAUSE HE HAS A DEFECTIVE CAPACITY FOR DEALING WITH CARBOHYDRATES.

William Banting found this out a hundred years ago and by applying the knowledge he lost nearly 3½ stones in a year, painlessly and without starvation, enjoying good food and good wine while he did it.

He learnt from his doctor that carbohydrate is the fat man's poison. Here is what he wrote:

For the sake of argument and illustration I will presume that certain articles of ordinary diet, however beneficial in youth, are prejudicial in advanced life, like beans to a horse, whose common ordinary food is hay and corn. It may be useful food occasionally, under peculiar circumstances, but detrimental as a constancy. I will, therefore, adopt the analogy, and call such food human beans. The items from which I was advised to abstain as much as possible were: Bread . . . sugar, beer, and potatoes, which had been the main (and, I thought, innocent) elements of my existence, or at all events they had for many years been adopted freely. These, said my excellent adviser, contain starch and saccharine matter, tending to create fat, and should be avoided altogether.

Banting included butter in his list of forbidden food. We now know that it may be taken freely without causing weight gain.

Who was William Banting? He was the fashionable London undertaker who made the Duke of Wellington's coffin.

He was a prosperous, intelligent man, but terribly fat. In August 1862, he was 66 years old and weighed 202 lb. He stood only 5 feet 5 inches in his socks. No pictures of him are available today, but he must have been nearly spherical.

He was so overweight that he had to walk downstairs backwards to avoid jarring his knees and he was quite unable to do up his own shoe-laces. His obesity made him acutely miserable.

For many years he passed from one doctor to another in a vain attempt to get his weight off. Many of the doctors he saw were both eminent and sincere. They took his money but they failed to make him thinner.

He tried every kind of remedy for obesity: Turkish baths, violent exercise, spa treatment, drastic dieting, purgation; all to no purpose. Not only did he not lose weight, many of the treatments made him gain.

At length, because he thought he was going deaf, he went to an ear, nose and throat surgeon called William Harvey (no relation to the Harvey who discovered the circulation of the blood). This remarkable man saw at once that Banting's real trouble was obesity, not deafness, and put him on an entirely new kind of diet.

By Christmas 1862 he was down to 184 lb. By the following August he weighed a mere 156 lb. – nearly right for his height and age.

In less than a year he had lost nearly 50 lb. and 12¼ inches off his waist-line. He could put his old suits on over the new ones he had to order from his tailor!

Naturally, Banting was delighted. He would gladly have gone through purgatory to reach his normal weight but, in fact, Mr Harvey's diet was so liberal and pleasant that Banting fed as well while he was reducing as he had ever done before.

What was the diet which performed this miraculous reduction? We have Banting's own word for it, in his little book *Letter on Corpulence*, published in 1864.

Here is what he ate and drank:

Breakfast: Four or five ounces of beef, mutton, kidneys, broiled fish, bacon or cold meat of any kind except pork. One small biscuit or one ounce of dry toast. A large cup of tea without milk or sugar.

Lunch: Five or six ounces of any fish except salmon, any meat except pork, any vegetable except potato. Any kind of poultry or game. One ounce of dry toast. Fruit. Two or three glasses of good claret, sherry or Madeira. (Champagne, port and beer were forbidden.)

Tea: Two or three ounces of fruit. A rusk or two. A cup of tea without milk or sugar.

Supper: Three or four ounces of meat or fish as for lunch. A glass of claret, or two.

Night-cap (if required): A tumbler of grog (gin, whisky or brandy with water but without sugar) or a glass or two of claret or sherry.

In terms of calories this diet adds up to the astonishing figure of 2,800. An average modern low-calorie reducing diet allows a meagre 1,000 calories a day. Incidentally, I know of no particular reason why salmon and pork should be excluded, except for the imprecise knowledge of the chemical composition of foods in the mid-nineteenth century. Certainly, there is no need for a Fatten-Easily to avoid them now.

There must therefore have been something other than calorie reduction responsible for Banting's weight loss. What was the secret?

In his own words: 'I can now confidently say that QUANTITY of diet may be safely left to the natural appetite; and that it is the QUALITY only which is essential to abate and cure corpulence.'

The diet was made up almost entirely of protein, fat, alcohol and roughage (or what is now called fibre), with, of course, the vitamins and mineral salts contained in these foods. Mr Harvey, who designed it, had realized that it is *carbohydrate (starch and sugar) which fattens fat people.*

This is the simple fact which explains Banting's highly satisfactory weight reduction on a high-calorie low-carbohydrate diet. Perhaps it was too simple, for in spite of the excellent book which he published at his own expense and in which he gave all the credit to his doctor, William Harvey, contemporary doctors refused to believe it. The public, particularly those who were overweight, were impressed however and many people followed his diet successfully.

Banting's name passed into the language as a synonym for slimming. But the principles of his successful diet were not understood in the 1860s and he and his doctor were ridiculed by the medical profession.

To appreciate just how remarkable it was for Mr Harvey to have designed this revolutionary and successful treatment for Banting's obesity, it is necessary to know something of the medical opinions current at the time.

In 1850 the medical profession in Europe had accepted the theory of a German chemist, Baron Justus von Liebig (1803–73), that carbohydrate and fat supplied the carbon which combined with oxygen in the lungs to produce body heat. In terms of this theory, carbohydrate and fat were

'respiratory foods' and the cause of obesity was believed to
be an over-indulgence in these: or as contemporary phrase-
ology had it: 'For the formation of body fat it is necessary
that the materials be digested in greater quantity than
necessary to supply carbon to the respiration . . .'

The principle of the treatment of obesity based on this
theory was to cut off as far as possible the supply of food
especially dietary fat, and to accomplish this the patient was
exhorted to establish 'an hourly watch over the instinctive
desires', i.e. was subjected to semi-starvation.

William Wadd had already advocated such methods and
right down to today, doctors have gone on slavishly copying
them in spite of the mounting evidence that they were unsatisfactory, at least from the patient's point of view, if not
from the physician's.

With this background of medical indoctrination on the
subject of obesity to which many doctors have succumbed
since, with far less excuse, William Harvey went to Paris in
1856 and attended the lectures of Claude Bernard (1813–78)
the great French physiologist.

He heard Bernard expound his new theory that the liver
made not only bile but also a peculiar substance related to
starches and sugars, to which the name glucose had been
given.

Relating this new idea to the already well-known ones
'that a saccharine and farinaceous diet is used to fatten certain
farm animals', and 'that a purely animal diet greatly assists in
checking the secretion of diabetic urine', Harvey did some
original and constructive thinking. This is how he put it:

That excessive obesity might be allied to diabetes as to its
cause, although widely diverse in its development; and that
if a purely animal diet were useful in the latter disease, a
combination of animal food with such vegetable diet as
contained neither sugar nor starch, might serve to arrest the
undue formation of fat.

Now in Harvey's time, biochemistry was in its infancy and physiology was only just emerging from the shadow of the Middle Ages, so he could not explain his theory of altered carbohydrate metabolism in exact chemical terms. But he could test it out in practice and it was at this point, in 1862, that William Banting consulted him. We have Banting's own description of the happy results of that meeting.

The subsequent history of William Harvey and his patient is interesting. It shows how social and economic influences and the desire to run with the herd, which is in all of us, can cloud scientific discoveries with compromise and in bringing them into line with orthodoxy can rob them of all practical value.

Banting published his *Letter on Corpulence* in 1864, privately, because he feared, not without reason as it turned out, that the Editor of the *Lancet*, to whom he first thought of submitting it, would refuse to publish anything 'from an insignificant individual without some special introduction'.

The same sort of objection deterred him from sending it to the *Cornhill Magazine*, which had recently carried an article, 'What is the cause of obesity?', which in Banting's view was not altogether satisfactory.

Banting's pamphlet attracted immediate attention and was widely circulated. The treatment he described was phenomenally successful. The 'Banting diet' then became the centre of bitter controversy.

No one could deny that the treatment was effective but having first appeared in a publication by a layman, the medical profession, which was just beginning to climb the social ladder and was very much on its frock-coated dignity, felt bound to attack it.

The diet was criticized as being freakish and unscientific. Harvey came in for much ridicule and vituperation and his practice as a surgeon began to suffer.

But the obvious practical success of the 'non-farinaceous, non-saccharine' (high-fat, high-protein, low-carbohydrate) diet called for some explanation from the doctors, and this was supplied by Dr Felix von Niemeyer of Stuttgart, whose name was associated with a pill containing quinine, digitalis and opium. German physicians were then very fashionable.

Basing his argument on the teachings of Leibig, Niemeyer explained Banting's diet as follows: Protein foods are not converted to body fat, but the 'respiratory foods', fat and carbohydrate, are. He interpreted meat as lean meat and described the diet in terms which today would mean that it was a high-protein, low-calorie diet with fat and carbohydrate both restricted.

Of course the diet which actually slimmed Banting was not like that at all. It was a high-fat, high-protein, unrestricted calorie diet with only carbohydrate restricted.

Harvey had allowed Banting to take meat, including venison, poultry and fish – with no mention of trimming off the fat – in quantities up to 24 ounces a day which gives a calorie intake of about 2,800 when the alcohol and other things he ate and drank are included.

Dr Niemeyer had effectively turned Banting's diet upside down and the day was saved for the pundits. Niemeyer's 'explanation' was eagerly accepted and 'modified Banting' diets, based upon this phoney explanation, found their way into the text-books for the rest of the nineteenth century.

While all this 'rationalization' of his diet was going on, William Harvey was feeling the cold draught of unpopularity with his colleagues and nine years after the publication of Banting's pamphlet he publicly recanted. He came into line with Dr Niemeyer and explained apologetically: 'Had Mr Banting not suffered from deafness the probability is that his pamphlet would not have appeared.'

Thus Harvey was able to continue his peaceful career as a respected ear, nose and throat surgeon. But Banting stuck to his guns and in 1875 published letters showing that obese people lost weight effectively and painlessly through eating large quantities of fat meat.

In spite of an almost total lack of scientific knowledge of the chemical composition of different foods, Banting remained true to the principle William Harvey had taught him: avoidance of starchy and sugary foods as he knew them.

He kept his weight down without difficulty and lived in physical comfort to the age of 71.

This distortion of a genuine discovery, based on original observation, to make it fit in with current theories has happened again and again in our history.

Ever since Procrustes cut off the feet of people who did not fit his bed, established authorities with narrow minds have employed the cruel weapons of ridicule and economic sanctions against people who challenged their doctrines.

To the student of psychology this is a commonplace, but it is a great brake on scientific progress.

The howl that went up against Harvey and Banting was nearly as loud as the one which greeted Freud's *Interpretation of Dreams* in which he pointed out the facts of infantile sexuality. This is hardly surprising when one considers how sensitive most of us are to criticism of our views on our pet subjects.

Among the many diets which followed the publication of Banting's pamphlet, every variation of the three main foods was tried but always with restriction of the total intake.

It seemed that in spite of the real value of Harvey's observations and Banting's application of them, nutritionists could not bring themselves to abandon the idea that to lose weight one must eat less. The principle derived from the law of conservation of energy (what comes out must go in) on the basis of which it was deduced that the energy intake (consumption of food) must exceed the energy expenditure when obesity is developing.

Of course this is perfectly obvious. A man can't get fat unless he eats more food than he uses up for energy. But it is beside the point.

The real question that needs answering about obesity is:

What is the cause of the fat man's failure to use up as much energy as he takes in as food? It could be that he is just greedy and eats more than he requires. It could also be *that although he only eats a normal amount, some defect in the way his body deals with food deflects some of what he eats to his fat stores and keeps it there instead of letting him use it up for energy.* In other words, Mr Fatten-Easily may have a block in his metabolism which Mr Constant-Weight has not.

It is curious that up to 1900, apart from Harvey and Banting, only one person had ever considered this alternative explanation for obesity. This was an eighteenth-century physician, Dr Thomas Beddoes.

In 1793, Beddoes applied the new theory of 'pneumatic chemistry' which had originated with M. Lavoisier's experiments in France and held that during respiration the lungs took in oxygen, combined it with carbon derived from the food and expelled it in the form of carbon dioxide.

Beddoes thought that the oxygen might go deeper into the body than the lungs and that obesity might be caused by its combining insufficiently with body fat. This would lead to fat accumulating instead of being burnt up for energy.

He attempted to remedy this supposed defect of fat metabolism by introducing more oxygen into the system – but with no good result.

His theory was easily disposed of by the redoubtable William Wadd, who remarked: 'Dr Beddoes remained so inconveniently fat during his life that a lady of Clifton used to denominate him the walking feather bed.'

So the views of William Wadd prevailed and, apart from the Banting interlude, semi-starvation has been the basis of the treatment of obesity in this country right up to the present day. Only the words have changed. 'Calorie control' has now replaced Wadd's 'taking food that has little nutrition in it'.

Within the principle of total food restriction, most reducing diets gave a high proportion of protein up to the year 1900. Then the American physiologist, Russell Henry Chittenden, published an indictment of protein, purporting to show that it was the cause of many diseases, and from that time obese patients were generally kept short of this vital food in their already short rations. (Lately, protein has been coming back into favour, and most of the current, popular slimming diets follow Niemeyer's modification of Banting. That is to say, they are high-protein and low-calorie, with fat and carbohydrate both restricted.)

There was the start of a break away towards more rational thinking on obesity with von Bergmann and the 'lipophilia' school. He, like Beddoes, suggested a diminished oxidation of fat and explored the metabolism of the obese for evidence of abnormality which could account for a special affinity for fat and an excess of storage over use.

The snag again – as with Beddoes – was the lack of any effective treatment to fit in with the theory.

Harvey had had an effective treatment with a theory no doctor would believe. Beddoes and von Bergmann had good theories but no treatment.

So as the twentieth century ran on into the thirties the view became more and more widely accepted that obesity was caused by an inflow of energy greater than the outflow, caused simply by careless over-eating and gluttony.

Popular books on slimming became mainly concerned with tricks for persuading people to eat less while seeming to allow them to eat more.

In 1930, Newburgh and Johnson summed the matter up thus in the *Journal of Clinical Investigation*: 'Obesity is never directly caused by abnormal metabolism but is always due to food habits not adjusted to the metabolic requirements'; i.e. over-weight never comes from a defective ability to mobilize fat from the fat stores but always from over-eating.

This appeared to be the last word and doctors and slimming 'experts' all over the world settled down to trying to persuade their obese patients to eat less.

With the 'obesity comes from over-eating' dogma enshrined

in history and hallowed by the blessings of the high priests of modern physiological research, imagine the impact on the medical world of the news in 1944, that cases of obesity were being treated effectively at the New York City Hospital with diets in which more than 24 ounces of fat meat was allowed a day. Patients were encouraged to eat to the limit of their appetites and some who were sceptical of the diet ate very copiously indeed. But they still lost weight.

The man in charge of this treatment was Dr Blake F. Donaldson.

At the time, Great Britain was still in the grip of severe wartime rationing and minimal amounts of fat and protein foods were obtainable. So this American revival of Bantingism was for the time being of academic interest only in this country.

But from that time onwards, unrestricted-calorie, high-fat, high-protein, low-carbohydrate diets for obesity were on the map again and in the United States at any rate they gradually gained in popularity.

Research workers in Britain were not idle, however. Many of them had been to America, and Donaldson's work and later Dr Alfred Pennington's caused great interest.

Then in July 1956, in *The Lancet*, Professor Alan Kekwick and Dr G. L. S. Pawan published the results of a scientific evaluation of Banting's diet undertaken in their wards at the Middlesex Hospital in London. They proved that Banting was right. Here is their conclusion: 'The composition of the diet can alter the expenditure of calories in obese persons, increasing it when fat and proteins are given and decreasing it when carbohydrates are given.'

This work had considerable impact on medical opinion and was widely mentioned in the press. Here is a quotation from the February 1957 number of the American journal, *Antibiotic Medicine and Clinical Therapy*:

Kekwick and Pawan, from the Middlesex Hospital, London, report some news for the obese. All of the obese subjects studied lost weight immediately after admission to hospital and therefore a period of stabilisation was required before commencing investigation.

If the proportions of fat, carbohydrate and protein were kept constant, the rate of weight loss was then proportional to the calorie intake.

If the calorie intake was kept constant, however, at 1,000 per day, the most rapid weight loss was noted with high fat diets . . . But when the calorie intake was raised to 2,600 *daily in these patients, weight loss would still occur provided that this intake was given mainly in the form of fat and protein.*

It is concluded that from 30 to 50 per cent of weight loss is derived from the total body water and the remaining 50 to 70 per cent from the body fat.

In other words, doctors now have scientific justification for basing diets for obesity on *reduction of carbohydrate* rather than on reduction of calories and fat.

Before going on it should be explained that Banting did in fact take some carbohydrate. Kekwick and Pawan and other investigators have shown that up to 60 grammes (just under 2 ounces) of carbohydrate a day are compatible with effective weight reduction on a high-fat, high-protein diet, although in some subjects even this amount will slow down the rate of weight loss. In such cases further restriction of carbohydrate with stricter adherence to the high-fat, high-protein foods results in satisfactory weight loss again.

Between 1957 and 1974 when he died, I saw Professor Kekwick from time to time, and Dr Pawan kept me up to date with their research on fat metabolism at the Middlesex Hospital. Kekwick was particularly interested in the physiological mechanisms controlling fat mobilization, concentrating most of his research as Professor of Medicine and Director of Clinical Research at the Middlesex Hospital in London, on the expenditure side of the energy equation (see p. 42, Chapter 2), enquiring into why some people, as in Professor Dodds's experiment, could automatically step up their expenditure of energy whenever they ate too much, so that their weight remained steady, while others could not do this and got fat instead.

He emphasized again and again that the fat cells all over the body behave as an organ and that they have a rich blood supply which enables them to enter into minute to minute changes in metabolism.

The idea that the adipose tissue in the body behaves as an organ is not new. It was first suggested in 1870, and ever since then, anatomists, physiologists and embryologists have returned to the idea. The fat organ is very large indeed, making up from one fifth to one quarter of the total body weight in normal people, and capable of increasing to over half the body mass in obesity. Most people think of adipose tissue as having a poor blood supply, probably because it is pale compared with muscle and because it bleeds little at operation. But research has shown that it has an extensive blood supply, laid out as a loose network of very small capillaries, and that the density of these tiny capillaries is greater than that in muscle, and second only to liver which is the most richly supplied organ in the body.

Kekwick said: 'It cannot be pretended that these ideas of the structure and function of the adipose organ will stand the test of all further investigations . . . it is only suggested that perhaps they are more nearly related to the true state of affairs than previously held views that fat exists as an inert calorie store. If so, adiposity becomes open to assault by different means than those previously employed.'

What he meant – and he told me this several times in conversation – was that once you get away from the input side of the energy equation and the boring business of totting up and trying to restrict calories, and look at possible ways of stepping up energy expenditure, a whole new field opens up in the treatment of obesity.

In 1957, Kekwick and his biochemist colleague, Dr Pawan, published a further paper showing that the type of food eaten influences the rate of fat mobilization from the fat organ, and they went on to investigate the various hormones known to increase the liberation of free fatty acid (the form in which fat circulates in the blood and supplies energy) from adipose tissue. They found that adrenaline, corticotrophin and growth hormone did this and they began looking at a substance extracted from the urine of fasting subjects, to which the name Fat Mobilizing Substance has been given.

In August 1960, the *British Medical Journal* published as its main article Kekwick's Bradshaw lecture to the Royal College of Physicians (delivered in London on 5 November 1959). It was entitled 'On Adiposity', and gave an account of all the research on obesity up to that time. In it he referred to Fat Mobilizing Substance (FMS) and gave a table of the conditions governing its appearance in human urine and another showing the effects of injecting it into mice.

It was concluded that people fasting or taking mainly fat and protein, produce this hormone from their pituitary glands and that in mice it mobilizes stored fat and causes weight loss. People taking a normal, mixed carbohydrate-rich diet do not produce it, nor do they make any on a low-calorie intake consisting mainly of carbohydrate. People with poor pituitary function do not make it either. It could be a very important hormone in the control of obesity, once it has been purified and made available for prescription, but it is likely to be expensive.

Professor Kekwick found that injected into mice, FMS produced loss of weight, the loss being mainly carcass fat and bearing some relation to the dose given. The food intake of the animals was the same as that for controls injected with saline. FMS also produced a rise in blood lipids, blood ketones and liver fat within six hours and was capable of liberating free fatty acids from an isolated pad of fat.

Four years later, in 1964, in a lecture on obesity to medical postgraduates at West Middlesex Hospital in Isleworth near London, Kekwick said that two pharmaceutical firms were making FMS and had enough to treat some humans, but that the injections were causing severe allergic reactions in experimental animals.

Since then, Dr Pawan has told me that this allergy hazard has been avoided by further purification and that teams of research workers in many centres besides his own are studying FMS and its effects: in Budapest, in Bordeaux, at Lafayette University in America and in London, Ontario. FMS is very unstable and is quickly decomposed by light, heat and oxygen, so that it has to be stored in dark ampoules after freeze-drying, and kept under nitrogen with an anti-oxidant added as a safeguard. It is being given to experimental human subjects by intramuscular injection, dissolved in water or saline, in 5 mg. doses. It mobilizes fat from the fat stores and causes weight loss in the obese, by stepping up energy output. Eventually it should become a means of converting a Fatten-Easily into a Constant-Weight.

I end this chapter with a quote from Kekwick's Bradshaw lecture:

The subject of adiposity is one of importance. It has been described as one of the major health hazards in modern life in the western world. Whether this be true or not, there is little doubt that people with enlarged adipose organs are unhealthy; that they die prematurely; that they are prone to diseases such as hypertension, diabetes, cholecystitis, and osteoarthritis; and that many of them are psychological cripples.

Public intolerance of this condition has never been so intense, as evidenced by the interest taken in this subject in almost every newspaper and magazine. This is in contrast to the somewhat resigned view taken by the medical profession of which Banting (1864) was complaining 100 years ago. Doctors too often tend to blame their long-term failure to relieve obesity on the gluttony of their patients. It is submitted that satisfaction with the too simple view that fat represents an inert calorie store has retarded and is retarding developments in this field.

In the next chapter the calorie-counting fallacy will be further examined, in the light of what we know of the evolution of man in relation to his diet.

References to Chapter 1

p. 15   Sir Charles Dodds's experiment with over-feeding people and
         showing that some could keep their weight steady was
         described in the *Proceedings of the Royal Society of Medicine*,
         1950, vol. 43, p. 342.

p. 16   Further experimental support for the idea that some people
         can automatically step up their calorie expenditure when over-
         fed, and thus avoid becoming fat, was furnished by some
         researchers at Guy's Hospital in London. Their summary
         was as follows: 'Food supplements containing 1,000 and
         2,000 calories were given nightly by tube to five young men
         and women for periods up to thirty-six days. They caused
         no suppression of voluntary food intake. Each subject's gain
         in weight was much less than would be expected from the
         calorie value of the food supplements.' Hunt, J. N., Ash-
         worth, N., Creedy, S., Mahon, S., and Newland, P., 'Effect
         of nightly food supplements on food intake in man' (from
         the Department of Dietetics and Physiology, Guy's Hospital,
         London, SE1), *The Lancet*, 6 October 1962, p. 685.

p. 16   These findings were confirmed in America by Miller, D. S.,
         and Mumford, P., in the *American Journal of Clinical
         Nutrition*, 1967, 20, p. 1212, who showed that some subjects,
         when deliberately over-fed, failed to gain the expected weight.

p. 16   The quotation from *The Times* medical correspondent is from
         the 11 March 1957 edition. More recently Professor John
         Yudkin has said the same sort of thing in the 1972 edition
         of his Penguin book *This Slimming Business*: 'Overweight
         comes from overeating. And overeating need not mean a lot
         of food, but too much food, which still may be relatively
         little.'

p. 22   Claude Bernard (1813–78) made the discovery that sugar
         (glucose) was made in the liver after a protein meal in 1855.
         He called the process 'internal secretion' and was the first
         to use this term.

p. 27   Ernst von Bergmann (1836–1907), a Berlin surgeon, is best
         known for introducing the steam sterilization of surgical
         instruments.

p. 28   Blake F. Donaldson, a New York physician who died in
         1963, published an account of his unlimited fat meat treat-
         ment of obesity, *Strong Medicine*, in 1960 (Doubleday, New
         York; Cassell, London, 1962).

p. 30   The subject of the fat organ, and the evidence for its inte-
         grated behaviour as an organ, was reviewed in 1940 by

Wells, H., *Journal of the American Medical Association,* *114,* pp. 2177–2284.

p. 31   Kekwick and Pawan's 1957 paper in *Metabolism,* 6, p. 447, showed that the type rather than the amount of food eaten influences the rate at which fat is mobilized from the fat organ.

p. 31   The first publication from Kekwick's team at the Middlesex Hospital on Fat Mobilizing Substance (FMS) was in Chalmers, T. M., Kekwick, A., Pawan, G. L. S., and Smith, I., in *The Lancet, 1,* 1958, p. 866.

p. 31   Kekwick's 1959 Bradshaw Lecture 'On Adiposity' was published in the *British Medical Journal,* 1960, *2,* pp. 407–414.

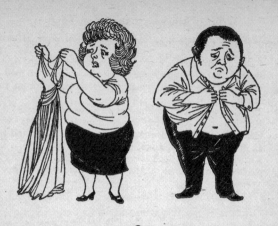

2

The Calorie Fallacy

Before going any further, it is important to be sure of the meaning of some of the words we have been using: fat, protein, carbohydrate, and calorie.

Fat, protein and carbohydrate are names for the main chemical classes of which foods are composed. When someone says that a food is fat and protein most of us visualize an egg or a steak and when they say fat and carbohydrate, we think of bread and butter or biscuits or cake.

Since the rise of dietetics as a branch of popular science, many people have learnt enough about the chemical composition of common foods to say roughly how much fat, protein or carbohydrate they contain.

This is essential knowledge for anyone wishing to Eat Fat and Grow Slim, for without it you cannot avoid carbohydrates, nor can you choose the high-fat, high-protein foods.

To help you decide exactly about the composition of any particular food, there is a list of all the common foods at the end of the book, in Appendix B, in which the proportions of fat, protein and carbohydrate are given. From this you can make up your own menus of permitted foods, or check on the composition if you are eating out.

The beauty of this method of slimming is that once you have got the hang of the proportions of fat, protein and carbohydrate in the foods you choose to eat, *you can afford to ignore calories altogether*. For as Banting so wisely said: 'Quantity of diet may be safely left to the natural appetite. It is *quality* only which is essential to abate and cure corpulence.'

The much publicized diets with emphasis solely on calories are fallacious. *It is excess carbohydrates and not calories only that make a fat man fat*. The tiresome business of totting up daily calories, on which most modern reducing diets are based, is a waste of time for an obese person. Because a fat man may maintain his weight on a low-calorie diet, if it is taken mainly as carbohydrate, but he will lose weight on a much higher calorie diet *provided he eats it mainly in the form of fat and protein*.

What is a calorie?

The calorie is the unit of heat. Just as inches are units of length and pounds or grammes are units of weight, calories measure the amount of heat (and therefore energy) a particular food will provide.

One gramme of fat provides 9 calories.
One gramme of protein provides 4 calories.
One gramme of carbohydrate provides 4 calories.

All food, of whatever sort, provided it can be digested and absorbed from the gut, can be used to give heat and energy for muscular movement and the various internal processes of the body.

The steam engine analogy holds good this far.

*

Theoretically, the amount of heat (number of calories) that can be provided by any particular bit of food is the same whether it is burnt in a steam engine, the human body or a special laboratory oven called a calorimeter. The one exception to this is protein which is not burnt quite as completely in the body as in the calorimeter.

But in obesity, the *kind* of food more than the *amount* determines the extent to which it is burnt or stored as fat. The proportion of calories obtained from carbohydrate is more important than the total calorie intake. Some people cannot get used to the idea of the body burning food to give itself heat and energy. 'Where does the burning take place?' they ask.

Well, of course, there are no flames, but obviously since the body maintains a constant temperature even on a cold day, heat must come from somewhere and combustion of a sort does occur in every cell in the body just as it does in a pile of grass mowings left at the end of the garden.

The most astonishing thing about protoplasm, which is the living basis of every cell, plant, animal or human, is the way in which, without any apparent effort, it is able to carry out chemical processes which could not be performed even in the largest and most modern laboratory.

It does it by means of complex chemical substances called enzymes, which the body has evolved over aeons of time. These enzymes are highly specific to the jobs they are designed to do and they are handed on from parents to children in the genetic code carried on the chromosomes in the nuclei in the protoplasm of every cell in the body. We tamper with these enzyme systems at our peril.

The word 'enzyme' means, literally, 'in yeast', because they were first discovered in yeast cells which use them to convert sugar into alcohol in wine-making. Louis Pasteur was the scientist involved.

To convert fat, protein or carbohydrate molecules into

energy as they are presented to the cells by the blood stream, requires long chains of enzymes which depend for their integrity on the proper nutrition of the body as a whole. Fats and proteins can provide the building blocks for their construction. Carbohydrates cannot. All animal life depends on these enzyme systems. They are the very stuff of our existence.

The light flashing at the end of a firefly's tail involves chemical processes more intricate than those going on in the atomic piles at Harwell. Dr Edward Staunton West, Professor of Biochemistry in the University of Oregon Medical School, Portland, USA, emphasizes this point in the introduction to the 1956 edition of his text-book of Biophysical Chemistry, which deals with the chemistry of human metabolism:

One of the most marvellous things about protoplasm is the efficiency of its chemical processes and the mildness of the conditions under which they take place. Food materials are synthesized and organized into definite kinds of highly complex protoplasmic structures in an aqueous medium of nearly neutral reaction and at body temperature. Carbohydrates and fats are rapidly and completely oxidized, under the same mild conditions, to carbon dioxide and water with the liberation of as much energy as if they had been burned in oxygen at the temperature of an electric furnace. Here in protoplasm we have chemical reactions proceeding quite differently from those commonly observed by the chemist in his test tube. The main reason for the difference is that the chemical processes of living things are largely controlled by catalytic systems known as enzymes which are highly specific in their actions.

Nevertheless in spite of the qualitative differences between the chemistry of an engine and of the human body, the same basic reaction takes place whenever or wherever there is combustion with the evolution of heat:

Coal + Draught =
Smoke + HEAT → Steam → Movement

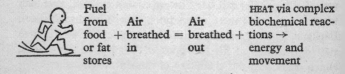

Basic equation   CARBON + OXYGEN = CARBON DIOXIDE + HEAT

Fuel from food or fat stores	Air breathed in	Air breathed out	HEAT via complex biochemical reactions → energy and movement

Here the steam engine analogy with the human body should properly end, but most slimming pundits press on and argue that it is your calorie intake, or total consumption of food *alone*, which determines whether you gain or lose weight. Fat is often severely restricted because it is the most concentrated source of calories.

On 23 June 1968, *The Observer* published in its colour magazine an article on weight control, with advice from Dr H. Beric Wright, Consultant to the Institute of Directors' Medical Centre in London – a pretty high-powered chap. They took a stout director-type named Harvey Martin, aged 41, and showed a picture of him tucking into an expense-account lunch. Here is what they wrote about him: 'How many calories does he consume a day? His diet chart for a week averages about 2700 a day. And how many does he use up in his daily activities? About 2500 – a net surplus a week of around 1400. The crux of weight control balance is that if you eat as many calories as you use up, your weight will remain steady. If you eat more you will gain weight, and if you eat less you will lose weight. How can the weight-conscious Mr Martin tell which way the calorie is crumbling?'

Sounds reasonable, doesn't it? And pretty simple too. Just the sort of reasoning that would appeal to a bunch of directors, many of whom are accountants. The trouble is that it is not the whole story. It may be true for the obesity or leanness of a bank balance but it is not always true for the human body, as I hope to show.

The crux of weight control lies in something not mentioned in the statement just quoted. It is, of course, perfectly obvious that if you eat more calories than you use up you will gain weight. But to take the bank balance analogy a stage further, what about deductions before he can take his money out? Bank charges, PAYE, even a bit of embezzlement by the bank staff. Mr Martin's body could turn up its built-in thermostat and burn off a lot of his daily 2700 calories, and then if he kept up the same amount of physical work and exercise, he might even lose weight on this generous intake. But Dr Wright does not seem to consider this possibility. He presses on with his profit and loss argument: 'If he keeps this up,' said Dr Wright, 'he will be putting on weight at the rate of 1 lb. of fat every five weeks; 1 lb. of water makes it double – say 10 lb. a year.'

In other words, if my mathematics are right, by the time he is 61 and nearly ready to retire, he will have put on 15 stone! As he weighed 15 stone 9 lb. at 41, he will then top the scales at over 30 stone – ready perhaps for a new career as the fat man at a circus, and all on quite a normal food intake by any standards: 2700 calories a day – about the same number that enabled Banting to slim.

Of course even a non-medical person knows from his own observation that this progressive and massive gain in weight rarely takes place, even in a Mr Fatten-Easily eating carbohydrate. At some point, as I shall show in Chapter 6, a fat man's excess weight levels off and his metabolism gets him back into calorie equilibrium on the same food intake that has fattened him, although at a higher weight than he should be for his height, build and age.

It is curious and depressing to see how medical slimming 'experts' persistently ignore the expenditure side of the energy equation:

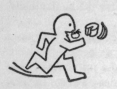

Calories in, as food	=	Calories put away as fat	+	Calories burned up in the body
(A)	=	(B)	+	(C)
INTAKE		STORAGE		EXPENDITURE

By assuming that all foods of whatever kind are treated alike by the body in terms of calories-for-energy, and that the fat stores are inert dumps with no life of their own, doctors like Beric Wright can do their sums and predict a quite exceptional weight gain for people like Harvey Martin. But the human body is not a machine. It is a living, self-regulating organism of great complexity, and as Professor Kekwick has shown (Chapter 1) the fat organ is one of the most active organs in the body, with a rich blood supply, and it enters into the minute-to-minute supply of energy both from carbohydrate and fat. It also organizes storage. Its functions in the energy equation are as important as those of the liver – perhaps more so.

So there is nothing really surprising, looking at the energy equation again, in finding that B and C can vary independently of each other and make nonsense of the calorie-counting routine.

A Fatten-Easily on quite a small intake of mainly carbohydrate food could take it straight to his fat stores and a metabolic block could prevent him getting it out again for use. If he were on a low-calorie diet this would mean he was actually semi-starving while getting fatter. On the other hand, if he took a normal number of calories mainly in the form of fat and protein he might stimulate his fat organ to disgorge some of its stored fat and his metabolism to burn it up by increasing his production of heat and radiation and evaporation from the skin. This would burn up not only the food he was taking in but even some of his stored fat also — so he would actually lose weight on a larger number of calories than made him gain on starch and sugar.

A machine like a motor car or a steam engine cannot do this, a living organism with a nervous system, hormones and enzymes can and does. This is what makes physiology and medicine more interesting than engineering.

Anyone who has followed the argument so far can see that the calorie-counting approach to obesity is over-simple and unsatisfactory. It assumes that the body treats all kinds of fuel alike and that once you have overstepped your calorie ration for the day, the excess is laid down as fat whether the fuel is fat, carbohydrate or protein. Fat is considered to be the most fattening food because its calorie value is greatest.

We now know that the calorie value of fat is irrelevant as far as slimming is concerned, and that fat is the *least* fattening of all foods because, in the absence of carbohydrate, it (and to a lesser extent protein) turns the bellows on the body fires in a fat person and enables him to mobilize his stored fat as well as helping him to burn up the food he eats more efficiently. On a high-fat diet, water accounts for 30% to 50% of the weight lost. (The other 50% to 70% comes from body fat.)

Turning the bellows on the body fires makes all parts, including its largest organ, the skin, work harder. This gives rise to a considerable increase in the insensible loss of water from the skin surface and to a subjective feeling of warmth. Fat people on high-fat diets often remark on this.

Insensible or 'dry' perspiration is water which evaporates from the skin without appearing as beads of sweat. It has no smell.

We all lose water in this way all the time, but when a fat person's metabolism is stimulated by a high-fat diet, this insensible perspiration increases in proportion to the rise in the metabolic rate, and contributes to the weight loss.

To go back to the steam engine for a minute: the orthodox, 'it's-all-a-matter-of-cutting-down-the-calories' boys talk as if a fat man's engine is stoked by a robot fireman, who swings his shovel at the same pace whether fat, protein or carbohydrate is in the tender.

This is true for Mr Constant-Weight, but as he does not get fat anyway, it is only of academic interest to us. It is certainly not true for Mr Fatten-Easily, with whom we are concerned. Mr Constant-Weight has a robot stoker in his engine. The more he eats – of whatever food – the harder his stoker works until any excess is consumed so he never gets fat.

Recent research has shown that Mr Fatten-Easily's stoker is profoundly influenced by the kind of fuel he has to shovel. On fat fuel he shovels fast. On protein slightly less fast but on carbohydrate he becomes tired, scarcely moving his shovel at all. His fire then burns low and his engine gets fat from its inability to use the carbohydrate which is still being loaded into the tender. Mr Fatten-Easily's stoker suffers from an inability to deal with carbohydrate, but he *can* work fast on fat and protein.

So why not feed him fat and protein, cutting out the carbohydrates? That way you spare him the calorie-counting, which is awfully tedious, and turn him into a Mr Constant-Weight.

What is it that causes Mr Fatten-Easily to be affected by carbohydrate in this way while Mr Constant-Weight can deal with all foods alike and burn up any excess automatically, like the robot stoker?

The answer to this question has only recently been found and it is one of the keys to obesity. Biochemists and physiologists have discovered that Mr Fatten-Easily's inability to deal with carbohydrate is due to a block or diversion in the chain of chemical reactions leading from glucose to the release of heat and energy in his body.

Glucose is the form in which most carbohydrate is absorbed from the gut. Every bit of starchy or sugary food we eat has to be broken down by our digestive enzymes to glucose or other simple sugars, before it can be taken out of the gut and into the body for use. Once through the gut wall, the glucose, in solution, is carried in the blood along veins leading to the liver. What is not wanted for immediate conversion to heat and energy is stored in the liver as a complex sugar called glycogen and further storage can take place by changing glycogen into fat.

In Mr Constant-Weight these chemical changes go smoothly and rapidly, and are reversible, i.e. the fat can quickly be broken down again to give energy and, by stepping up his internal combustion, Mr Constant-Weight soon burns up any excess carbohydrate he has eaten, thus keeping his weight steady.

The chemical reactions which enable the body to deal with food in this way are extraordinarily complicated and we know that they can go wrong. We also know that they depend on certain hormones and enzymes which some people may lack or be unable to manufacture properly.

It is this lack, or deficit, which is thought to distinguish the Fatten-Easilies from the Constant-Weights, who can deal with an excess of carbohydrate by fanning their metabolic fires until the surplus is consumed.

Feed a fat man fat and protein in place of starch and sugar and he will deal with that quite well, drawing on his stores of body fat in the process. Paradoxically, he will eat fat and grow thinner. He will also feel well because he will no longer be subjecting his body to starvation and he will be tackling the fundamental cause of his obesity which is *not* over-eating but a defect in the complex biochemical machinery of his body.

The question: why has Mr Fatten-Easily got this defect? is an interesting one which can best be answered by looking at man's evolution and adaptation in relation to his diet.

If you discount the allegorical, Old Testament story of instant creation, then the evolutionary theory of man's development from his humble unicellular beginnings is the only one that holds water.

It is based on the archæological evidence of the rocks, with their petrified fossil remains, on Darwin's work on isolated communities of animals which he visited during the voyage of *The Beagle*, and on the remains of ape-like and human-like creatures dug up by researchers like Leakey in Africa and Lewis in India.

Most scientists now accept that the first primates – man's hominid ancestors – separated from their ape-like stock about twenty million years ago. This is a long time, but not nearly as long ago as the first oxygen-using animals, the trilobites, which fed on marine plants and on each other 500 million years ago. Their fossilized remains can be seen today in the Cambrian Welsh Hills, formed when the earth's crust folded and brought them up out of the sea.

Before these trilobites, little spiny, spade-shaped creatures not more than four inches long, with eyes and antennae, the first known forms of life existed about 2000 million years earlier and have left their remains in the black flints of Ontario. These were the blue-green algae, some early fungi and a little one-celled organism with a flagella or whip-like appendage which it used to move around in the sea. Before that, the evidence of the rocks is silent, although recent research has suggested that bacteria or microscopic germs may have existed even earlier. But how did life itself originate in these very primitive forms?

The current theory is that life started on earth through the action of ultraviolet light, and other radiations from the sun, on a sort of primordial soup of simple chemicals. Free oxygen did not exist then, but hydrogen was present in large quantities. Oxygen was there all right, but combined in water, sulphates, phosphates, carbon dioxide and other compounds. Without free atmospheric oxygen to shield it, the earth's surface was bombarded by intense radiation from the sun. It has been shown experimentally that irradiation of a soup of simple chemicals such as existed on earth in those days leads to the spontaneous formation of amino-acids, the chemical building blocks of the protein constituents of protoplasm.

Amino-acids are the biochemicals still used to make living creatures today – including man – so here, over two billion years ago, you had the formation of the complex organic chemicals needed to make nucleic acid and other genetic cellular material. At what point these newly formed and increasingly complex organic chemicals came alive and formed themselves into self-repairing and self-reproducing systems is still a mystery. But it must have happened somehow or we would not be here today.

Most people think of life as some isolated miracle, but chemists and astronomers now believe that it is no accident and that given the right mixture of chemicals and exposure to radiation such as permeates outer space, the creation of life is inevitable and may have occurred and be occurring in galaxies other than our own.

On earth, the first creatures with backbones, the fishes, evolved 300 million years ago during the Devonian period, at which time the earth's crust began to fold and form mountains. Early plants had begun to spread, and some grew to great size, the ancestors of the little horse-tails still found in our fields and hedgerows, and mined as coal in the pits. These primitive trees grew in huge swamps and soon became infested with insects, among them the first cockroaches, which appeared 250 million years ago.

Large reptiles evolved from the fishes and came out of the sea to feed on the rich vegetation. Some grew to a great size, up to eighty feet in length, weighing sometimes over fifty tons. From among these herbivors the first reptilian carnivors developed and held sway until the age of the dinosaurs came to a sudden end during the Cretaceous period 100 million years ago. Why did this happen? Some people say it was due to sudden climatic change or to a tilting of the earth's axis, but it is more likely that these creatures ran out of vegetation and thus out of phosphorus with which to grow their huge bones. Perhaps this was the first instance of an imbalance between a population and its food supplies.

After the dinosaurs became extinct a change occurred in the vegetation: seed-bearing plants took over from the earlier pollen-bearers. Within the next thirty million years all the orders of mammals evolved, including the predecessors of man: the lemurs and tarsiers which preceded the monkeys and apes. At this point a significant division of evolutionary style took place: the cats, mammoths and horses going for muscle and brawn, the lemurs, monkeys and apes developing bigger and better brains and nervous systems.

Today man, with his highly developed nervous system, has taken over the planet and the bulky, muscular animals are very much on the way out, remaining mainly by human permission, as domesticated animals or in game reserves, so that we see an exploding population of humans – over 3000 million of them – with but a handful of large mammals in the wild state. Looking back at evolutionary history, it is quite possible that man himself could go the way of the dinosaurs unless he can come to terms with the crisis in his food supplies and environment in which he suddenly finds himself.

Part of the crisis is that of adaptation to a modern, Westernized diet, and if we do not solve it quickly by changing the way we produce and market our food, we may deteriorate in Europe and America to the point where others, with a more primitive diet, take over. Already the writing is on the wall for all who can look beyond the glib assurances of the politicians that we have never been better fed. Consider the ominous signs:

(1) An ever-increasing epidemic of degenerative disease of the heart and blood vessels, manifesting as coronary thrombosis and strokes, which are affecting our people at a younger and younger age;

(2) Massive increase in the incidence of diseases of the digestive system: hiatus hernia, gastric and duodenal ulcer, gall bladder disease, regional ileitis (Crohn's disease), appendicitis, colitis, cancer of the large bowel, diverticulitis and piles;

(3) More and more cases of diabetes, particularly the maturity-onset type;

(4) More mental disease;

(5) More dental disease;

(6) More obesity;

(7) More allergy;

(8) More low-weight babies with mental sub-normality. (This was stated by Professor Raymond Illsley of the Medical Research Council's Medical Sociology Unit in Aberdeen, and reported in *The Times*, 23 May 1974.)

(9) More rheumatism.

Why should all these things be happening to us at a time when we are supposed to be prosperous and never better fed?

And how on earth could all these diverse maladies have a single cause in what we are doing to our food? The answer lies in our history and the evolution of diet since our pre-human ancestors branched off from the apes in the rain forests, came down from the trees and emerged on to the grasslands as animal-hunting bipeds with highly developed brains and nervous systems.

There is a case for saying, as Stefansson did, that the

change from a vegetarian, gatherer's diet to one of animal meat and fat determined the change from apehood to manhood.

During the two to three million years that man has walked upright, he has been a hunter for nine-tenths of that time, subsisting on infrequent, large meals of animal tissue. Only in the last 6000 years has he eaten a high-cereal diet and only in the last 100 years, a diet high in refined starch and sugar and increasingly contaminated with chemical additives – substances made in the laboratory and never presented to the body chemistry before. Is it surprising that our bodies and brains, evolved as they were on natural fat and protein, are now showing adaptive breakdown in the face of new foods with which they are not equipped to deal?

Man comes at the end of mammalian evolution. His nearest rivals are all dying out and he has been left on top thanks to his highly-developed and specialized nervous system. The brain and the nerves are made very largely of structural fats, unsaturated fats called phospholipids, and of proteins, few of them able to be synthesized from simpler chemicals in the body. All these essential fats and proteins must be provided ready-made in the diet. So man has evolved as a predator.

Looking at the earliest predators, some of the single-celled organisms which ate other single cells to acquire complex molecules which they could not make for themselves, we can see the advantages of such a way of eating. It makes room on the cellular genetic tapes for further specialization if you scrub off the instructions for making a complex vitamin like B_{12} by eating the B_{12} in a simpler cell which has made it for you.

So too with man the predatory meat-eater. Instead of getting the unsaturated fats and proteins essential for the building of his brain by laboriously collecting seeds, insects and green shoots, he eats the flesh of a herbivor which has already made these essential substances from plant food, and in one mouthful gets more brain-food than he would in a day's gathering in the forest.

This is how the idea of 'essential' foods came in. Whilst algae can make all their own nutrients from the simple salts and other chemicals dissolved in the water in which they float, more than 40% of the components of our cell membranes and nervous system must come from food – and the best and most concentrated source is other animals, fishes and birds.

So man must have essential fats and proteins, with their essential amino-acids, in his diet if he is to grow a good nervous system and arterial tree, and keep them in good shape into old age. The importance of dietary fat, especially the unsaturated fats which contain essential fatty acids which the body cannot make for itself, is now generally recognized. It is now known that these essential fatty acids are important for the formation of the newly discovered hormones called prostaglandins which have a wide range of effects on many tissues: on smooth muscle contraction, blood pressure and the nervous and reproductive systems. Essential fatty acids are also involved in normal skin metabolism and may play a part in preventing degenerative changes in the white matter of the brain and thus in the prevention of diseases like multiple sclerosis and presenile dementia, in which the nervous system goes wrong before the rest of the body.

What we are seeing more and more today is a rise in degenerative diseases of all kinds due to our taking a diet poor in essential nutrients and high in useless carbohydrate fuel, refined and contaminated with additives to the point where our enzyme systems are clogged and poisoned. Hence, in large part, the strokes, coronaries, digestive disorders, brain damage and deterioration, and, of course, obesity which is nothing more than a result of presenting to the body unsuitable calorie-laden carbohydrate food in unwieldy amounts at frequent intervals.

What the fat person needs is infrequent meals of first-class protein and essential fats, foods on which his ancestors evolved millions of years ago and which Mr Fatten-Easily can

metabolize smoothly, without waste, using the efficient biochemical machinery which he has inherited from the Stone
Age.

Besides a variable assortment of essential unsaturated fatty
acids (depending on how the animal is fed) most animal fats
marketed and eaten today contain predominantly saturated
fatty acids, and on a diet low in carbohydrate these are the
principal source of energy for use in muscles and the maintenance of body temperature.

Vegetable oils, except those of coconut, palm, cashew nuts
and cocoa beans, are rich in essential, polyunsaturated fatty
acids, so too are the fats and oils of fish and poultry.

To end this chapter on the calorie fallacy, I want to quote
a part of the foreword to the earlier version of this book, by
that great surgeon and medical writer, the late Sir Heneage
Ogilvie. It is as true today as when he wrote it in 1957:

Fat is the caloric reserve material of nature. The whale stores
fat in his subcutaneous layers, against the rigours of life at
the Pole, the camel stores it in his hump against hard times
in the desert, the African sheep stores it in his tail and his
buttocks against the day when even the parched grass shall
have withered away.

But fats are more than stores of reserve caloric material.
They are heat insulators, they are fillers of dead spaces, and
they are facilitators of movement in rigid compartments such
as the orbit [eye socket], the pelvis and the capsules of joints.
They are also essential building materials. Animal fats contain
three groups of substances: the neutral [saturated] fats which
are chiefly energy providers, the lipids containing phosphorus
[the unsaturated fats] that enter into most tissues and bulk
largely in the brain and the central nervous system, and the
sterols [like cholesterol] that are the basis of most hormones.
The body must have proteins and animal fats. It has no need
for carbohydrates, and, given the two essential foodstuffs, it
can get all the calories it needs from them.

The statistician looks on nutrition as a matter of calories
and on obesity as a question of upset caloric equilibrium.

A calorie is a unit of heat, a unit of potential energy, but not a unit of nutrition. Fellows of the Royal Society and doctors with political leanings, talk of calories as if the human body were a machine requiring a certain amount of fuel to enable it to do a certain amount of work.

A motor-car needs calories, and we give it calories in the form of petrol. But even a Rolls-Royce cannot find its own fuel. It cannot separate motor spirit and lubricating oil from the crude mixture brought by tanker from the wells of Kuwait. It cannot clean its own pipes, clear its own choked jets, grind its own valves, re-line its own bearings when they are worn, and replace defective parts as they need renewal. The body can do all these things, but to do them it needs food not fuel.

References to Chapter 2

p. 46   Darwin, C. R., *On the Origin of the Species by Means of Natural Selection*, New York, 1860
On the origins of man, see also two books by Robert Ardrey, *African Genesis* (1961) and *The Territorial Imperative* (1967), Fontana Books.

p. 51–2 Fat metabolism and the role of saturated and unsaturated fatty acids in the body have been reviewed by Dr G. L. S. Pawan in *The Practitioner*, April 1974.

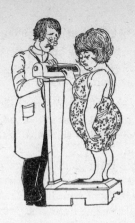

3

The Anti-Starch and Sugar Doctors
—the Clinical Evidence

Four Centuries BC, Hippocrates, the father of medicine, wrote:
'Let your food be your medicine and your medicine your
food.' Hippocrates said that corpulence is not only a disease in
itself but the harbinger of others. Aristotle echoed this when
he wrote: 'Fat persons age early and therefore die early.'
So, intelligent, good observers in ancient Greece were already
warning people of the dangers of obesity.

When the great Græco-Roman civilization collapsed and
barbarism took over in Europe, medical interest in obesity
seems to have been lost in the struggle for survival under
squalid, unhygienic conditions, and it was not until the middle
of the nineteenth century that doctors had enough peace
and prosperity in England to use their growing scientific
knowledge and curiosity in the investigation and reappraisal
of the causes of overweight. This is where Harvey the ENT
surgeon came in with his patient, Mr Banting (1806–76). (See
Chapter 1.)

In 1872 Harvey published his paper 'On Corpulence in Relation to Disease – with some remarks on diet'. On pages 99 to 101 of this monograph, he wrote:

> The treatment of obesity would now seem to rest upon a more sure basis than it has hitherto done, the investigations by Dr Dancel having been somewhat instrumental in leading to this result.

> In proof of the truth of this remark we may look back for a moment to the curative agents formerly in use. Thus we find a tolerable list of remedies in the pages of Maccary, which includes – bleeding from the arm or jugular vein, leeches to the arms, dry cupping, prolonged blistering, vegetable diet with vinegar, acids (except nitric and phosphoric), hot baths, salt water baths, baths of Aix, Spa, Forges, Rouen, and occasional starvation, decoction of guaiacum and sassafras, scarifications, salivation, grief and anxiety to be induced, purgatives, issues, pricking the flesh with needles, walking with naked feet, and removal of exuberant fatty tissue with the scalpel. Since this ridiculous catalogue was published, Turkish baths, sea-voyages, very little sleep, emetics, digitalis, soap (a relative of Mr Wadd's ordered a quarter of a cwt. of Castile soap for his own eating), salt, mercury to salivation, the inhalation of oxygen gas, purgatives, diuretics, the extract of the fucus vesiculosus, and preparations of bromine or of iodine have been freely tried.

> But all these plans, however perseveringly carried out, fail to accomplish the object desired, and the same must be said of simple sobriety in eating and drinking.

> The explanation of all this is very simple. Food consists of azotized or nitrogenous and non-nitrogenous principles. The *former* – the nutritive* or plastic class – includes all

---

* Of course Harvey was not aware that structural fats, with their essential fatty acids not synthesizeable in the body, are essential nutrients. However he did, accidentally, allow Banting plenty of them when he let him eat unlimited meat, fish and poultry.

fibrous and albuminous matters, such as animal food; these matters aiding the formation of blood and muscle, but not entering into the composition of adipose tissue. The *latter* – the calorifacient or respiratory class – consists of oily and fatty matters, with sugar, gum, starch, and vegetable acids, all of which contain carbon and hydrogen, the elements of fat. Man undoubtedly requires a mixed diet; that is to say, nitrogenous food is needed for the formation or renewal of the tissues and other nitrogenous parts of the body; while the respiratory food is required for the production of the fatty components of the body, and as affording materials for the respiration and the production of heat. Hence it is clear that while we may limit the non-azotized substances, they must not be altogether cut off. Moreover, it is of practical importance to remember that the elements which are chemically convertible into fat are rendered more fattening if alcoholic liquids be added to them in the stomach, probably because of the power which stimulants possess of lessening or delaying the destructive metamorphosis.

These arguments of Harvey's are about a century ahead of their time – in fact we are only just catching up with them today.

Other doctors at the time seem to have agreed with Harvey, for he went on:

Wadd has also told us that 'among the Asiatics there are Brahmins who pride themselves on their extreme corpulency. Their diet consists of farinaceous vegetables, milk, sugar, sweetmeats, and ghee. They look upon corpulency as a proof of opulence, and many arrive at a great degree of obesity without tasting anything that has ever lived.'

Dr Fothergill stated that a strict vegetable diet produces exuberant fat more certainly than other means.

Notice that Harvey classes 'oily and fatty matters' with the sugars and starches as 'calorifacient' (=heat-producing) foods. He did not know the difference between structural fats and obesity or storage fats, but he was certain that the surest way to put on weight was to eat a high-starch diet. In fact, the diet which he prescribed for Banting, as I have already pointed out in Chapter 1, was what we would now call high-protein, high-fat and low-carbohydrate, with no calorie restriction.

In Banting's day, nearly all the animals were free-range so that their fat was more unsaturated then than it is now as a result of battery farming and intensive feeding of stalled animals. It is interesting that Harvey makes the distinction between 'oily and fatty matters', sensing perhaps that they are different: the oils being mainly what we now call unsaturated and the fats hard and saturated. However that may be, it is certain that with his high consumption of meat, fish and fowl, Banting took a lot of good, essential, unsaturated fat and that this contributed to his general sense of well-being as well as to his weight loss.

Before leaving Harvey, I want to give his summing up, which I think is absolutely on the ball:

Farinaceous and vegetable foods are fattening, and saccharine matters are especially so. The instance of slaves in Italy, who got fat during the grape and fig season, has been quoted by Galen. In sugar-growing countries the negroes and cattle employed on the plantations grow remarkably stout while the cane is being gathered and the sugar extracted. During this harvest the saccharine juices are freely consumed; but when the season is over the superabundant adipose tissue is gradually lost.

The necessity of abstaining from the saccharine materials and all those allied to them, which in the metamorphosis of digestion form sugar, will be obvious from what has been stated.

We now move on to another pioneer in the proper understanding of obesity: Dr Francis Hare, an Australian physician
and expert on alcoholism, who came to work in England and
published his two-volume book *The Food Factor in Disease*
in 1905. He had been consulting physician to the Brisbane
General Hospital and Inspector General of Hospitals for
Queensland.

Hare was not primarily interested in obesity – although he
talks about it.

His book is mainly about the understanding and treatment
of the whole range of disorders commonly associated with
obesity: angina, high blood pressure, circulatory, kidney and
other degenerations, bilious attacks, catarrh, etc. Like Surgeon
Captain Cleave at the present time (see Chapter 6) he lumps
all these ailments together as having a single cause which
he terms 'hyperpyraemia' – by which he means, as does
Cleave, the presentation of too much concentrated carbohydrate fuel, sugar, in unit time to the liver and the rest of
the body.

Here is how Hare defines hyperpyraemia (Volume I,
page 3): 'accordingly, it was determined . . . to adopt pro-
visionally the hypothesis that carbonaceous material might,
in certain circumstances, accumulate in the blood to an ultra-
physiological degree, such accumulation constituting a primary
cause of pathological action. To the blood state supposed to
eventuate, the term hyperpyraemia (Greek: *pyreia*=fuel)
was applied.'

At the end of Volume II (pages 393–4), he gives his conclusions. These are very like those of Harvey, Kekwick,
Pawan, and Cleave, and all those who subscribe to the metabolic view of obesity and its associated disorders:

From the standpoint of practical medicine, preventive and
curative, the most generalised conclusion to be drawn from
the theory of hyperpyraemia is, I think, that we cannot any

longer afford to ignore 'the stoking of the engine'. Seeing that the capacities of the individual for physiological management of his fuel supply are widely variable, the intake of fuel will have to be graduated more accurately than heretofore to his capacities, not less than to his seeming necessities: it will have to be graduated to his capacity for digestion and absorption, to his capacity for regulating the income (perhaps here inversely in many cases), to his capacity for expenditure from the blood, whether by katabolism (*breaking down*), anabolism (*building up*) or direct loss. [Taken together, anabolism and katabolism are termed metabolism. – AUTHOR]

So already, by the turn of the century, some reputable doctors were suggesting that obesity was not just a simple result of over-eating, and its cure just a calorie-cutting exercise, but a more complicated matter concerned more with the kind of food you eat than the amount, and involving differences in metabolism between one person and another. Starches and sugars were already being incriminated and the fat person's inability to burn up as much food as he takes in was being looked on in the light of growing insights into physiological mechanisms. Ever since then, right up to the present day, seventy-five years later, the evidence for the rightness of this metabolic view has grown stronger and stronger, thanks to the work of other doctors and scientists who, like Harvey and Hare, were not afraid to go against establishment thinking.

Next in my line of pioneers in this respect comes Dr Blake Donaldson, a Scottish physician who practised in New York and who startled the medical pundits in 1924 by slimming fat patients and curing their complications, including arthritis, high blood pressure and heart disease, with a diet of unlimited fat meat, water, an occasional baked potato in its jacket, and black coffee.

I visited him twice, in his New York office, first in 1958 and subsequently in 1963, shortly before he died, and can vouch for the loyalty of his patients and the good results they achieved under his guidance.

In 1962, Donaldson came to visit a wealthy patient in London and I was able to tape-record an interview with him at the Berkeley Hotel, where he liked to stay. He was a fairly formidable man but with great charm and a relaxed way of talking. He had just written a book about his methods (*Strong Medicine*, published by Doubleday in New York and Cassell in London).

Here is part of that interview:

Dr M.: When and how did you come upon the ideas which led you to write your book?

Dr D.: About 1919. I was faced with the problem of people with heart disease, fat people who were short of breath, had swollen feet and could not lose weight.

I tried them for a year on a low calorie diet, with a very bad result. At the end of the year practically none had lost weight, they were all breathless and had swollen feet.

I decided to try something new. I went to the American Museum of Natural History and consulted the Curator there and asked him what the teeth of the people were like in the old days. Because, as you know, all the cells in the body at first have common qualities, then they specialize afterwards.

If you can find the best food for teeth, to prevent holes in the teeth, you have perhaps got the best foods for stomachs and hearts and everything else.

So I wanted to see what teeth were like in the dawn of history. They showed me skulls from the old Eskimo burial grounds; people who lived on nothing but caribou meat and the walrus, essentially fat meat, and they were astonishingly good teeth.

It occurred to me that it might be the primitive nature

of the food that prevented dental caries, and I came away from there determined to try primitive foods as a basis for any sensible way of taking weight off fat people with heart disease.

Dr M.: This was when you first came out of the Army?

Dr D.: Yes.

Donaldson was looking for a job at that time and heard that Dr Robert Halsey, the famous heart specialist, wanted an assistant to rent his office in the afternoons and help run his cardiac clinic at the New York Postgraduate Medical School. He offered Donaldson the job.

Donaldson accepted gladly and rented a bedroom on the East Side where he paid little rent but had to stand the legs of his bed in kerosene tins to keep the bed bugs off.

He set to work among Halsey's heart patients, poor people mainly, visiting them in their homes and getting to know them well.

Halsey had impressed on him two basic facts: (1) that almost nothing is known about what is normal; and (2) that all cells in the human body have primary qualities in common and only specialize later.

Donaldson thought that the cells of which we are made might have common nutritional needs.

The same food that keeps teeth healthy might prevent cataracts developing in the eyes, and might also be good for the cells involved in the mysterious diseases like duodenal ulcer, migraine, high blood pressure and obesity.

He put the idea up to his chief who advised him to go ahead and try it in the heart clinic.

Dr M.: How long was it after starting this idea that you made it routine and based your whole practice on it?

Dr D.: Well, of course, in those days we were very much frightened that if you ate meat alone you would get something called acidosis (now called ketosis); that the meat was just too acid and needed starch to neutralize this acid.

With a good deal of fear and trembling I gave these fat cardiacs nothing whatever but fresh meat without salt, and potato (as a compromise to the idea that you would get acidosis if you did not have some starch), and a cup of coffee.

I found that many of them lost weight beautifully at the rate of 7 lb. per month. But there were others who did not lose. So again with considerable fear and trepidation we tried cutting out the potato and just gave them meat and coffee. And apparently we struck something that was of great practical value. We found out the patients could live on just fresh meat and a cup of coffee three times a day and lose weight at the rate of 3 lb. a week (you don't want to lose weight much faster than that, otherwise the skin becomes wrinkled).

But it takes many years to prove that people won't develop acidosis if they just live on fresh fat meat and coffee, so that forty years have gone by and in that time I have only struck two families (and there were several members in each family) who developed an odour of dead violets on the breath (acetone) when they lived on nothing but meat, and they felt weak and dizzy, the symptoms we ordinarily associated with acidosis. So these people were not allowed to lose weight rapidly. They had to lose weight gradually, and they were told to eat grapefruit. This cleared up their symptoms and they lost weight at the rate of 7 lb. per month.

Now we are fairly convinced that flour is the root of all evil. It's too concentrated a food.

Mind you, when you make such an arbitrary remark as that you want to remember that there are 20% of people who can eat and drink anything and maintain a normal weight, feel fine, reproduce their kind and live a normal span of years.

But it is the other 80% in which we are interested. There

are a great many of us who get overweight or develop many of these unpleasant symptoms when we eat flour.

Dr M.: After they've improved and lost their overweight, have you tried reintroducing these patients to flour on a test basis to see whether their obesity comes back?

Dr D.: Yes. And every time I've failed to show that they can tolerate it. The moment flour is introduced their weight goes right up again.

When you reduce their weight to normal you have to prove their weight can stay normal; that's very important. You have to get them thin enough so that they can eat four things with a meal and show no gain in weight. They have to be able to eat fat meat, with salt and potato, with butter and raw fruit, a full cup of coffee three times a day and show no gain in weight.

Dr M.: And they may have unlimited quantities. There is no restriction on the amount?

Dr D.: No, there is no restriction on the amount.

Dr M.: How many patients over the last forty years have you treated on this basis?

Dr D.: About 17,000. I now have a group of about 1500 patients over the age of 75, who from five to forty years have avoided flour and have kept primitive food as their basic way of maintaining health.

Dr M.: This is what I call a Stone Age diet. Would you agree with that description? It is a pre-cereal diet.

Dr D.: Well, I should say that it is perhaps 6000 years old and twenty years ahead of its time. I think this will be a popular idea in twenty years; that flour is a bad thing for about 80% of the population.

Dr M.: And do you also ban all carbohydrate derivatives – sugar, chocolate, etc.?

Dr D.: Once you have a fat person under control you reduce that person's weight to normal. I find that I am unable to feed them sugar in any form and unable to feed them flour and unable to give them more than one alcoholic drink in twenty-four hours and unable to keep them under control unless they take a thirty-minute walk before breakfast.

Dr M.: What is the significance of this thirty-minute walk before breakfast?

Dr D.: I wish I knew. We're fairly sure that after you walk for ten minutes without stopping before breakfast bile begins to drain and in the next twenty minutes you drain a pint. We're fairly sure that you increase elasticity in your arteries when you take a thirty-minute walk before breakfast.

Dr M.: Have any records been made on the results achieved with these 17,000 patients of yours?

Dr D.: They keep coming to see me!

In another part of the above interview, not reproduced here, Donaldson mentioned that Dr Pennington had worked in his office for a time. So it is convenient to take him next.

The late Dr Alfred Pennington, of Delaware, New Jersey, spent most of his working life as consultant physician to the Medical Division of du Pont, the American chemical concern.

Soon after he joined them he was given the task of slimming the firm's overweight executives, who found it difficult to stick to low-calorie diets while entertaining clients.

After sifting through the medical literature, and talking to Donaldson, he decided that obesity is caused by an inability to utilize carbohydrate food for anything except making fat. He was very successful with the du Pont staff, and as a result received a lot of (to him) unwelcome publicity in the American women's magazines.

When I visited him in 1958 just before his death I found him still practising what he preached. We had an all-meat lunch at his house. He was a lean and upright figure with a keen intelligence, and a most kindly way with him. Like Donaldson, he was a cardiologist.

He told me that most of his twenty du Pont executive

patients had high blood pressure when he began to slim them on an all-meat diet of around 3000 calories per day. By the time their weights had returned to normal their blood pressures had come down to normal too.

Idiopathic hypertension (high blood pressure of unknown cause) is one of the commonest of the so-called 'stress' disorders of the civilized world. Millions are crippled by it every year and it is a common precursor of strokes and coronary thrombosis. I believe it to be a disease of maladaptation to specific foods.

Pennington alleviated it in his du Pont executives at the same time as he reduced their excess weight, on a diet which eliminated all starch and sugar (cereal foods) while allowing unlimited quantities of fat meat.

Both Donaldson and Pennington were tall, lean ectomorphs, probably unworried by personal weight problems. My next doctor is very different, inclined, like me, to endomorphy and obesity.

Dr George L. Thorpe of Wichita, who to the best of my knowledge is still alive, is a delightfully ebullient mid-Westerner who had paid his way through medical school in the thirties by hopping with his guitar from one-night stand to one-night stand in a jalopy of an aeroplane – a sort of medical Burl Ives.

I talked with him at the Annual Meeting of the American Medical Association in Minneapolis in 1958.

At the previous Annual Meeting in 1957 in New York, Thorpe had been Chairman of the Section of General Practice and had made the cereal-elimination approach to overweight the subject of his address from the Chair.

Thorpe hates to call his method a diet. 'Proper eating is the normal and complete answer to the problem of excess weight,' he said. 'The words diet and dieting should be avoided.'

Thorpe told me that several years ago, while he was

considering a personal problem of excess weight, it became evident that huge numbers of calories in his daily total came from three to four large glasses of milk, two to three bottles of soft drinks, numerous slices of bread, and an educated taste for cookies, candy, and sweets in general, all of which are concentrated carbohydrates. Cereal grains, historically, were cultivated in order that limited agriculture areas might supply food to support population densities not otherwise possible. They are concentrated forms of food, readily assimilated by the body, containing small residue of bulk, and so may be eaten in quantities far in excess of the calorie needs, without sensation of fullness. All carbohydrate foods and most drinks fall into this category, either by virtue of their origin or the reaction of the body to them. Milk is actually a liquid infantile food, the use of which man has carried over into his adult life and which, in general, satisfies the definition of concentrated carbohydrate.

The simplest to prepare and most easily obtainable high-protein, high-fat, low-carbohydrate diet and the one that will produce the most rapid loss of weight without hunger, weakness, lethargy or constipation is made up of meat, fat and water. The total quantity eaten is not important, but the ratio of three parts of lean to one part fat must be maintained, as any decrease in the fat portion will reduce the weight loss.

Black coffee, clear tea and water are used without restriction. Reduction of salt, while not required, will increase the speed of weight loss.

So far, all the modern doctors I have quoted have been American and to show that there are good European doctors thinking and working along the same lines, I want to end this chapter with references to my friend and colleague Dr Wolfgang Lutz, of Salzburg, Austria (whose book *Life without Bread* gives great support to the Eat-Fat-Grow-Slim argument), and to a British Consultant Physician, Robert Kemp, TD, MD, FRCP, whose book *Nobody Need be Fat* is well worth reading.

Robert Kemp has long been interested in the clinical and metabolic aspects of obesity. He is Physician to the Walton and Newsham Hospitals in Liverpool.

In 1967, he edited a symposium on obesity and nutrition, published in *Medical News Magazine*. Here is part of what he wrote in his editorial:

The last twenty years have been increasingly concerned with the problems raised by the over-plentiful diet. Indeed we have now broken through at the other extreme to discuss the acaloric diet [*no-calorie diet*] and the use of prolonged fasting as a form of treatment [*see Chapter 6, where fasting is discussed*]. Nothing could illustrate more aptly the paradoxical problems of Western civilization. Dietetic abuse is now the current theme, though this is no novelty in medical history.

Criticism is directed a little uncertainly towards animal fats and perhaps more convincingly towards excess of carbohydrate. Whereas the calorie was of some theoretical use in measuring insufficient diets, it has almost no practical value in trying to fix a nutritional ceiling for the individual. Moreover the calorie makes no distinction as to source. It may equally come from fat, protein or carbohydrate, though the illness may well call for a careful choice . . . We know enough now to be fairly certain that a full menu is likely to bring us just as many patients as did the previous scarcities, so that the distinction between gourmet and gourmand may yet become a matter of everyday clinical significance.

And that is what this book is all about. That it is useless in treating obesity to count calories only. What you eat (gourmet) is much more important than how much (gourmand or glutton).

At the end of his article in the same symposium, Dr Kemp ums up as follows: 'Clinical study of overweight patients aises three points. Firstly, there is the obesity-prone meta-olism [*Mr Fatten-Easily*] or the absence of protective lean-ess [*Mr Constant-Weight*]. Secondly, the almost invariable ver-indulgence in carbohydrate. Thirdly, there is the patient's mazing tolerance of an unpleasant and dangerous state for what may be the best part of a lifetime before coming for reatment [*see Chapter 6 below for the psychiatric aspects of this*]. It is this third point which gives obesity the status of a disquieting problem. It is for this reason that we have o much active untreated disease, so many defaults and elapses in treatment and such a flood of ultimate complica-ions into the hospital wards.'

Finally – Dr Lutz. In his book *Lieben ohne Brot* (Life without Bread), which I am hoping one day to finish trans-ating so that it may find an English publisher, he gives some onvincing personal testimony of the efficacy of a low-arbohydrate, free-calorie diet. Here is what he says in the ection headed 'Trying it out on myself':

I was forty-five years old when, in March 1958, I began to cut out carbohydrates from my diet. Up to then I had, for several years, suffered from a painful arthrosis of both hip joints that caused me to limp quite noticeably.

The X-ray pictures showed considerable deformation of the joints and this was by no means a minor complaint. My general fitness had been decreasing. Three hours of hard office work was all I could manage without becoming completely exhausted. At the end of my working day I used to have a strange sensation of weakness in my arms and legs as though the muscles were not working properly. As soon as I arrived at the conclusion that only by returning to the nutritional habits of our ancestors would people be able to overcome the diseases of civilization, I changed

abruptly to a diet that was almost 100% free of carbohydrate. Here is the menu which I followed for the first
two years:

Dr Lutz's low-carbohydrate, high-fat, high-protein, free-
calorie diet:

Breakfast: Half a cup of heavy cream coffee without sugar.
Midday meal: Soup (bouillion, mushroom, asparagus) prepared without flour, possibly with an egg or marrow;
7 to 11 ounces (200 to 300 grammes) of meat, often rather
fat; vegetables prepared with butter, but without flour.
Dessert: cottage cheese, cream, etc., with little sugar, an
omelet with fruit preserves or stewed fruit (again with very
little sugar, or better without any), possibly cheese with
butter, black coffee with cream.
Evening meal: 7 to 11 ounces (200 to 300 grammes) of meat
with vegetables, or cold meat cuts (all-meat sausage, etc.),
cheese with butter without bread, one bottle of beer.

As far as alcohol is concerned, I am not overly strict. As
long as you are careful to restrict carbohydrates, you may
be fairly generous with alcohol.

The transition to a diet mainly consisting of meat was
a smooth one. I found I had to go to bed a little earlier
but I felt more cheerful in the mornings. After about eight
months, the pains in my hips lessened and the limping
ceased.

My mental state also improved. I worked faster and was
bothered less by doubts and indecision. Consequently, I was
able to keep a brisker pace when dictating and taking
X-ray pictures. Thus I gained time for my hobbies, which
I had abandoned one by one as I had had hardly enough
strength for my professional work. My heart does not act
up with palpitations any more, as it used to do in moments
of stress. My temper too has improved markedly. I have

become a happier, more balanced individual and I no longer feel depressed.

With regard to weight, I have always been lean. Before the change of diet I weighed 143 lb. (65 kg.) at a height of 5 feet 11 inches. My muscles were poorly developed and my posture bad.

During the first year on the new regime, I lost about 2 lb. (1 kg.), but after this my weight increased slowly to 176 lb. (80 kg.) and finally settled down at a steady 154 lb. (70 kg.). This makes me well filled-out but by no means a corpulent person. Apparently my muscular system (and perhaps the calcium content of my bones?) has grown in strength and weight.

This is pretty impressive evidence from a doctor of the benefits of going back to a Stone Age type diet. Notice that Dr Lutz, who is an ectomorph, actually put on weight, but not too much, when he cut out carbohydrate. Further evidence of differences in the metabolism of fat and thin people.

With such obvious benefits accruing to people who cut out starch and sugar and eat lots of fat and protein, it is surprising that so many objections to high-fat diets have been raised. In the next chapter I shall deal with these objections and show how ill-founded they really are.

References to Chapter 3

p. 59   Hare, Francis, *The Food Factor in Disease* (2 vols.), Long
        man Green and Co., London, 1905.

p. 68   See also: Kemp, Robert, 'On metabolic and treatment aspect
        of obesity', *Practitioner*, 1963, *190*, p. 358, and 1966, *19*
        p. 358.

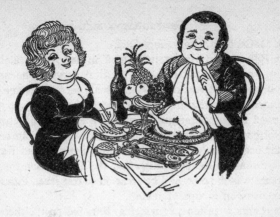

4

Objections to High-Fat Diets and the Anthropological Evidence

So far, I have given the historical, evolutionary, metabolic and clinical evidence for the effectiveness of high-fat, high-protein, free-calorie and low-carbohydrate diets in obesity. The evidence is pretty impressive and very widely based, but one serious objection must already have occurred to the reader in these days of soaring prices for meat and fish: the cost.

There is no doubt that the sort of diet which slimmed Banting is a lot more expensive than a modern, supermarket-based high-carbohydrate diet to which the majority of town dwellers in the West have become accustomed. With ingenuity, and by juggling with the cheaper dishes and menus given in Appendix C, it is possible to keep the cost down a bit, but if meat, fish and poultry prices rise much further, they will make the Eat-Fat-Grow-Slim approach to overweight impossible for all but top-income people, cowboys, butchers, fishmongers and farmers. So is there a cheaper alternative? I think there is, and I am going to call it the McCarrison/High-Fibre Diet.

Sir Robert McCarrison, who died in 1960 aged eighty-two, was a doctor in the Indian Medical Service who made some important observations on diet some forty years ago.

Besides an interest in diseases endemic to India he was impressed by the difference in physique and health between the Northwest Frontier tribes – Sikhs, Pathans and Hunzas – and the people of the plains: Madrassis, Bengalis and Kanarese. He came to the conclusion that the main reason for the difference was the diet, and he went on to test seven different Indian diets on groups of rats.

His results were most convincing. Rats fed on the diets of the hillmen, based on fresh stone-ground grain, milk, pulses (peas, beans and lentils), meat, fresh vegetables and fruit, did very well indeed. Of one group of rats maintained on this sort of diet for over five years, McCarrison wrote: 'They suffered no case of illness, no deaths from natural causes, no maternal mortality, no infant mortality.'

Rats on the Madrassi, Bengali or Kanarese diets did very badly. They did not grow well, and though they received the same care and handling as the other groups, their health was poor and they died early, particularly of respiratory and digestive disorders. Madrassis and Bengalis eat polished, processed rice from which most of the protein, fat, vitamins and mineral salts have been removed in the milling. They drink little milk, eat almost no meat and few fresh vegetables. They like sweets, particularly the women, many of whom are grossly overweight.

In one significant experiment, McCarrison fed rats on a typical late-1930s English working-class diet of white bread, margarine, sweet tea, boiled cabbage, boiled potato, tinned meat and tinned jam. 'Not only were the rats badly proportioned,' he reported, 'their coats lacked gloss, they were nervous and apt to bite their attendants, they lived unhappily together and by the 60th day of the experiment, began to kill and eat the weaker ones among them.' Not too unlike the behaviour of some people in the over-crowded and poorly-fed ghettos in our big cities today.

Obesity is very common among Indian plains-dwellers, when they can get enough to eat, whereas it is almost unknown among the people of the hills. So what was the essential difference between the diets which produced such strikingly different results on related groups of humans and rats? The Hunza or Pathan diet is whole and fresh and has been grown on healthy soil. The Madrassi or Bengali diet has had most of its wholeness removed, leaving just the white starch. It is not eaten fresh and is grown on poor soil. Another important difference is that all the fibre or roughage has been removed from the plainsmen's rice, while the hillmen, who use only stone-grinding, get plenty of bulky fibre. Hence my name for it: the McCarrison/High-Fibre diet.

For some years now, in England, there has been a McCarrison Society for doctors, dentists, vets and nutritionists, and I have been a member almost since the beginning. The society exists to propagate McCarrison's findings and to convince Government agencies and the public at large that faulty nutrition is the key to much of the ill-health and degenerative disease in Britain today. In 1971, Peter Bunyard, science editor of *World Medicine* (8 September 1971), reported on the first full-scale . conference of the McCarrison Society which met at Tekels Park in the Surrey countryside near Camberley, to discuss a strategy for sound nutrition.

Here is what Dr Barbara Latto, a Reading GP, said about the cost and content of a McCarrison/High-Fibre diet for good, positive health and the prevention of obesity:

Eating the 'right' kind of food need be no more expensive than eating processed foods, claims Dr Barbara Latto, secretary to the McCarrison Society, and a nutritionist. She has laid down some simple guidelines to what she considers to

be a good, cheap diet, the essentials being that the food must
be whole and fresh and whenever possible known to have
been grown on a healthy soil.

Daily: Plenty of whole-wheat bread and whole cereals,
such as whole-wheat soaked for 24 hours, brought to boil and
simmered for one hour. Milk, yoghurt, or cream, fresh or
dried fruit that has been soaked, and a little honey can be
added. Or the cereal can be eaten warm with cheese and herbs
and vegetables.

Only brown rice should be eaten and plenty of raw
vegetables as salads. Dairy produce is also important and in
addition to milk Dr Latto recommends cheeses and home-
made yoghurt.

White flour and white or brown sugar are to be avoided as
much as possible. Confectionery, including biscuits, pastries,
cakes, and sweets are out. They must be replaced with wholemeal bread and fruits. Bran is also a very good addition to
the diet.

By 'bran', Dr Latto means natural, unprocessed bran with
wheat germ, the material which is removed from the wheat
in the milling when white flour is made. It contains all the
most nutritious parts of the grain and is sold as feeding stuff
for animals such as pigs, who not surprisingly, in view of
McCarrison's experiments, do very well on it. The humans
who try to live on what is left, plus the additives the millers
put in, do less well.

Because it is, in a sense, a waste product of the milling
industry, natural unprocessed bran is cheap to buy, particularly in bulk, and I reckon that it costs about one penny per
week to give it daily to patients on my wards at the hospital
where I work. It cures not only constipation but also the faecal
incontinence which is the bane of nurses on long-stay, geriatric
wards. One to two tablespoonfuls, three times a day, mixed in
the food, will do the trick. It is quite palatable – like Bemax.

In the 22 December 1973 number of *The Lancet*,
Dr K. W. Heaton from the University Department of Medicine, Bristol Royal Infirmary, published an article explaining

how he thought a high-fibre diet helped to cure obesity. It is worth quoting his summary and introduction in full:

SUMMARY

Food fibre (or unavailable carbohydrate) provides three physiological obstacles to energy intake. (1) It displaces available nutrients from the diet. (2) It requires chewing, which slows down intake, especially of sugars, which, when freed of fibre, are soluble and can be drunk. Chewing also limits intake by promoting the secretion of saliva and gastric juice, which distend the stomach and promote satiety. (3) Fibre reduces the absorptive efficiency of the small intestine. The stripping of fibre, which occurs partially in the milling of white flour and completely in the refining of sugar, removes these obstacles. The refined products have an artificially increased energy/satiety ratio, increased ease of ingestion, and more complete absorption. Thus they are inherently liable to cause excess energy intake. The extreme commonness of obesity in Western countries may be related to the fact that most dietary carbohydrate is refined and fibre-depleted.

INTRODUCTION

Obesity is recognized as the 'commonest form of malnutrition' in our society, but the full extent of this malnutrition is greater than many realize. By the conservative definition of obesity as being more than 10% over ideal weight, roughly half the adult population of England is obese. Using stricter criteria, more than 90% of Scottish students carry more fat than the minimum which is probably the physiological optimum. Even these figures must underestimate the extent of overnutrition, since many people can ingest extra calories (especially as fat) without putting on weight. Overnutrition may be involved in the ætiology of such important and common diseases as diabetes, cholesterol-rich gallstones, and coronary-artery disease.

Is overnutrition inevitable in modern civilization? It may be if the theory that mechanisms controlling intake are inefficient at low-energy outputs is correct. However, this theory is by no means established, and alternative and less fatalistic answers to the question 'Why does civilized man

have such apparent difficulty in maintaining energy balance?'
must be examined.

It is widely assumed that overnutrition is the result of
taking an abnormal amount of food. Could it result merely
from taking an abnormal type of food? Little attention has
been paid to the changes in diet which have occurred with
the growth of modern Western civilization. There has been
a pronounced fall in the intake of starchy staple foods (mainly
cereals and potatoes), and a pronounced rise in the consumption of refined sugars. This is usually represented as a change
from complex carbohydrate (polysaccharides) to simple carbohydrate (monosaccharides and disaccharides). However, it
also involves a change from foods which were eaten whole
or only partly refined to foods which are highly refined.
Whole, unrefined plant foods contain their natural fibre intact,
whereas refined foods are invariably depleted of fibre.

The major sources of carbohydrate in modern Western
diets are white flour, which is very largely depleted of fibre,
and sucrose, which is wholly stripped of fibre (average daily
intakes in England 180 g. and 140 g., respectively). Carbohydrates are widely regarded as fattening, and carbohydrate
restriction is an integral part of almost all weight-reducing
diets. However, in primitive societies, where obesity is rare,
much more carbohydrate is eaten (for example, 580 g. per day
in rural Bantustan). This paradox may be explained by the
fact that in unsophisticated societies carbohydrate is eaten
with all or much of its fibre intact, as in home-pounded rice,
coarsely sieved maize, unprocessed bananas, and plantains.

I believe fibre to be a natural obstacle to nutrient intake,
and suggest that foods from which fibre has been removed
cause overnutrition, and that starch and sugar are non-
fattening when eaten with their natural complement of fibre.
This hypothesis developed from Cleave's concept of a
saccharine disease.

Cleave is Surgeon Captain T. L. Cleave, Royal Navy (retd),
who was formerly Director of Medical Research at the Royal
Naval Medical School at Alverstoke in Hampshire. In 1966,
after a lifetime of research into the diets and disease patterns
of people all over the world but mainly in India and Africa

he published his findings in a now famous book: *Diabetes, Coronary Thrombosis and the Saccharine Disease* (John Wright & Sons, 2nd ed., 1969). His co-authors were Dr G. D. Campbell, Physician to the Diabetic Clinic of the King Edward VIII Hospital, Durban, Natal, and Professor N. S. Painter, Hunterian Professor to the Royal College of Surgeons in London. Here is what they have to say about saccharine disease:

We consider that the correct name of the central disease referred to should be 'Refined-carbohydrate Disease', but because we ourselves dislike lettered abbreviations, such as 'RCD', and because the main refined carbohydrate involved is sugar, and the starch in white flour is converted in the body into sugar, we have, for ease in writing, made use of the term 'Saccharine Disease'. In this term we consider it essential that the word 'saccharine', meaning 'related to sugar', should follow the precept given by the *Oxford English Dictionary* and be pronounced like the river Rhine (as opposed to the chemical sweetener, which is pronounced sacchar*in* or sacchar*een*). The difference in pronunciation is the same as that between *shine* and *shin* or *sheen*. The term 'saccharine disease', pronounced as stated, is a convenient one, and even if it is not entirely acceptable, we suggest that it should be used until a better term is forthcoming.

Cleave's views on obesity are beautifully expressed by him in the chapter on obesity in his book, and they accord very well with the McCarrison view:

The type of obesity to be discussed here is the ordinary idiopathic or 'essential' type, and not those exceptional types associated with damage to, or tumours of, the diencephalon, or with disease of one of the 'target' endocrine glands. We consider that such obesity is one of the most obvious manifestations of the saccharine disease, the single primary cause lying in the consumption of refined carbohydrates. As already shown, the refining processes lead to unnatural concentration in the carbohydrates concerned, which deceives the tongue and the appetite, and leads to over-consumption – and this over-consumption is the sole primary cause of the over-weight. With unrefined, unconcentrated carbohydrates over-consumption does not occur, and obesity does not occur either, as we intend to demonstrate.

This line of reasoning positively excludes as a primary cause of obesity any fault in the instinct of appetite (such as the mysterious derangement postulated by some in a hypothetical 'appestat' centre in the brain); it likewise positively excludes as a primary cause any dislike of, and consequent abstention from, taking exercise. In short, it is advanced that, as regards obesity, the body, again, is not built wrongly, but is being used wrongly.

His attitude towards physical exercise is refreshing and encouraging to anyone who feels guilty about not taking the dog for a walk. Notice that he agrees with what Stefansson said to me about exercise in his letter (see Chapter 7, p. 151).

The view that obesity is due to insufficient exercise is just as vulnerable. In the first place, the lack of exercise held responsible is nearly always a *voluntary* lack, not an imposed lack. People are blamed for using lifts in office buildings and for not walking when they leave their offices. Yet this is what their natural inclinations often tell them to do. Some don't *want* to climb stairs, and don't *want* to go walking, either; they would rather sit down when they get home and put their feet up. Therefore, those who ascribe obesity to these instincts being wrong are just as vulnerable as those who ascribe it to the instinct of appetite being wrong, since they are open to the same critical attack. Throughout the whole animal kingdom, in fact, no living creature, unless forced to do so in order to get food, ever takes any more exercise than it wants to take. Nature obviously likes to conserve the heart – and certainly never inflicts on any organism the penalty of obesity for 'laziness'.

My three Dalmatians, who are fed a carnivorous meal once a day, and are not obese, take very little exercise apart from running into the garden to investigate a strange noise. When the family is not around, they spend nearly all the time curled up, asleep. Consider, too, Harvey's remarks on the uselessness of exercise and Banting's experience of rowing a boat on the Thames (see Chapter 7).

Here is Cleave on the exercise factor in rural and urban Zulus: 'The above figures show not only the remarkable freedom from obesity in the rural Zulus, but also the prevalence of it in the urban Zulus, especially the women. Although it is indisputable that differences in physical activity between rural and urban Zulus exist, we submit that any such differences could not possibly account for the supervention of obesity on such a scale. (And this quite apart from the fact that, for the reasons already given, we do not acknowledge lack of physical activity to be ever a primary cause of obesity, anyway.)'

Finally, Cleave's wholly admirable words on treatment:

From the argument presented above, it is clear that the treatment of obesity lies in the same fundamental step indicated in the other manifestations of the saccharine disease – the avoidance of refined carbohydrates. This treatment may be summarized in the case of obesity as 'seeking safety in dilution' – the dilution present in natural carbohydrates, through the existence of fibre. There are three points to be noted:

1. In the matter of the prevention of obesity, and in the early stages of the condition, the above is all that is required, but for established cases a certain amount of starvation will at first also be necessary, such as the omission of breakfast and afternoon tea.

2. Naturally desired exercise is encouraged, but forced exertions are not. The reasons for this have already been set out.

3. The authors have found that a careful explanation to the patient, of how Nature has been deceived in the production of obesity, is of the greatest assistance. An intelligent person,

looking around at the rest of creation, will recognize the truth for himself, and will then largely be in command of his own fate. It is, indeed, most advantageous that patients should have confidence in their own judgement in this way, rather than be obliged to accept edicts laid down by others.

Before going any further, I want to clear up an apparent contradiction which may be bothering some readers. I have strongly advocated a low- or non-carbohydrate diet of fat and protein in the first three chapters, and now, in an attempt to provide a cheaper diet I seem to have switched to quite a high-carbohydrate way of eating. I admit it looks funny, but I think there is a way of making both diets acceptable without abandoning any fundamental principles or being too devious.

Looking at the problem from an evolutionary and historical standpoint again: man must carry instructions on his genetic tapes for making the enzymes and hormones necessary for digesting and metabolizing all the types of diet with which he has had to deal for any length of time (by this I mean for millions rather than hundreds of years).

The two main types of diet we have been on are firstly the gatherer-type, monkey diet equivalent to a McCarrison diet, and secondly the all-meat, fat and protein diet I am advocating as the best for obesity. So although I think we function best on a Stone Age, all-meat diet, it is reasonable to say, as Cleave does, that man is an omnivor who can eat and metabolize practically any food that grows *provided it is unrefined and unprocessed*, with the natural fibre left in.

What we are *not* adapted to is the highly refined and unadulterated carbohydrate diet foisted on us by the food manufacturing industry in modern, urbanized society. And there is no reason why we should be adapted to artificial, concentrated carbohydrate because we have not been exposed to it for nearly long enough – one hundred years at most, which is but a fraction of a second in man's evolutionary day.

Anthropology, which is the study of different groups of

people in their native habitat, supports what I have just said absolutely and anyone who has travelled about the world can confirm that people manage to stay fit and a normal weight on widely different diets so long as those diets are whole and unrefined. As McCarrison said: 'The greatest single factor in the acquisition and maintenance of good health is perfectly constituted food.'

A baby born and reared on either a McCarrison diet or an all-meat diet will do well and not get too fat, particularly if it is breast-fed at first. But it is important that the parents even before conception should be on one or other of these good diets and absolutely vital for the mother to eat it during pregnancy, and while breast-feeding.

If, through faulty diet early in life, a child gets to be a fat adult, a period of starvation will be necessary as part of the slimming programme if McCarrison and Cleave diets are to be used, because they do not have a fat-mobilizing effect. I have quoted Cleave on fasting and agree with him except that he does not go far enough and advocate as I do a *total* fast for a week or two to get the weight loss going. All this will be developed in Chapter Six where fasting is discussed in more detail. It will also be touched on again in the final chapter, under 'prevention of obesity'.

So much for the moment for the cheaper way of slimming by means of the McCarrison/High-Fibre diet. Menus and suggested dishes and recipes are given in Appendices B and C, along with high-fat, high-protein dishes.

After high cost, the other five common objections raised are as follows:

1. 'High-fat diets are nauseating and make you bilious. No one could stick to such a diet for long enough to lose weight.'
2. 'High-fat diets cause ketosis and make you ill.'
3. 'High-fat diets may be all right in cold weather but they are too heating in hot weather.'

4. 'High-fat diets are unbalanced and cause deficiency
   diseases.'
5. 'High-fat diets cause heart disease.'

These seem to be reasonable objections, yet when we come
to examine them, we find that history, anthropology and the
highest medical and scientific opinion have refuted them.

1. High-fat diets are nauseating and make you bilious. No one could stick to such a diet for long

It is true that there are some people who suffer from complaints which make them unable to eat much fat. Gall-bladder
disease, by interfering with the flow of bile (necessary for the
digestion of fat), is the best-known example. Steatorrhoea,
another disease where the gut cannot digest fat, also requires
a low-fat diet. But these are *diseases* and the Eat-Fat-Grow-
Slim diet is not for people who are ill. It is for overweight
adults who are apparently healthy apart from their obesity.

First, then, what do we mean by a high-fat diet?

For the purpose of this book, it means a diet in which the
calories are derived mainly from fat and, if not from fat, from
protein.

Most people who eat meat consume about three parts of lean
to one part of fat because that is the palatable proportion. This
means that people who live *exclusively* on meat, derive about
80% of their energy from fat and the remaining 20% from
lean, because fat is a very much more concentrated source of
heat and energy than lean. Carbohydrate, as the glycogen
contained in meat, would amount to 1–2% of the calories.

In round figures the amount of food consumed would be
from six to nine ounces of lean meat and two to three ounces
of fat, cooked weight, at each of the three meals of the day.

Obviously, then, the people to study when we wish to
investigate the idea that high-fat diets are nauseating and
cannot be kept to for long, are those who eat nothing but
meat.

There are many such people, but let us take the Eskimos

irst because nearly everybody knows, or thinks they know,
omething about them.

The greatest authority on the Eskimo was Dr Vilhjalmur
Stefansson, the distinguished anthropologist and explorer. In
906, Stefansson revolutionized polar exploration by crossing
he Arctic continent alone, living 'off the country' on a diet
omposed only of meat and fish, travelling exactly as the
Eskimos did.

Not only did he remain in good health, but he enjoyed his
ood, ate as much as ever he wanted and did not put on weight.

More important from the slimming point of view, he never
aw a fat Eskimo. Here is what he says:

Eskimos, when still on their home meats, are never corpulent
– at least, I have seen none who were. Eskimos in their
native garments do give the impression of fat, round faces
on fat, round bodies, but the roundness of face is a racial
peculiarity and the rest of the effect is produced by loose and
puffy garments. See them stripped, and one does not find
the abdominal protuberances and folds which are so in
evidence on Coney Island beaches and so persuasive against
nudism.

There is, however, among Eskimos no racial immunity to
corpulence. That is proved by the rapidity with which and
the extent to which they fatten on European diets.

In other words, Eskimos stay slim on a high-fat diet, but as
oon as they start eating starch and sugar they get fat.

The European brings obesity to the Eskimo in addition to
is other 'gifts' of civilization.

So much for Eskimos who have never lived on anything
ut fat and protein. What about people who go on to an all-
meat diet after they have been used to an ordinary mixed
liet of cereals, sugar, vegetables, etc., as well as meat?

The key word here is pemmican, the most concentrated
ood known to man. It is made from lean meat, dried and
ounded fine and then mixed with melted fat. It contains
thing else.

It was originally the food of the North American Indian and, by adopting it, the early fur traders and pioneers were able to perform great feats of endurance.

Pemmican has been called the bread of the wilderness, but this is a romantic not a scientific description. Real pemmican is half dried lean meat and half rendered fat, by weight.

A man working hard all day on a meat diet needs a ration of six to seven pounds of fresh lean meat and a pound of fat.

Most authorities agree that this is equivalent to two pounds of pemmican and on this ration David Thompson, the British explorer, tells us in the Narrative of his Explorations in Western America 1784–1812 that men could slave at the hardest labour fourteen and sixteen hours a day, often in sweltering heat, as when paddling canoes up swift rivers and carrying their loads on their shoulders across portages (up beside rapids and over steep escarpments).

What happens when a European first eats pemmican? Does it make him sick? Can he eat enough of it to keep himself going?

George Monro Grant, D.D., LL.D. (1835–1902), in his book Ocean to Ocean, published in 1873, describes his experiences as secretary to Sir Sanford Fleming, on an overland expedition from Toronto to the Pacific doing preliminary work for the extension of the Canadian Pacific Railway.

Dr Grant was educated at Glasgow University and was ordained a Minister of the Church of Scotland. From 1877–1902 he was Principal of Queen's University, Ontario, where he gained a great reputation in education and politics. His personal experience of pemmican lasted not more than five weeks, but on the journey he travelled with a number of Europeans who had used it much longer.

The main value of Grant's observations is that they were made at the time, in diary form, not in retrospect. On page 24 of the London, 1877, edition he says: 'Our notes are presented to the public and are given almost as they were written so that others might see, as far as possible, a pho raph of what we saw and thought from day to day.'

After leaving Fort Carlton on their way up the North
askatchewan to Edmonton, Grant's entry for 19 August
872, says:

Terry gave us pemmican for breakfast, and, from this date,
pemmican was the staple of each meal. Though none of us
cared for it raw at first, we all liked it hot . . .

Pemmican and sun-dried thin flitches of buffalo meat are
the great food staples of the plains, so much so that when
you hear people speak of provisions, you may be sure that
they simply mean buffalo meat, either dried or as pemmican.

August 22: At the camp, the Chief treated them with
great civility, ordering pemmican, as they preferred it to
fresh buffalo.

August 26: Camped before sunset within twenty-seven
miles of Edmonton, and in honour of the event brought out
our only bottle of claret. As we had no ice, Terry shouted
to Souzie to bring some cold water, but no Souzie appearing
he varied the call to 'Pemmican.' This brought Souzie, but
great was his indignation when a bucket was put into his
hands, instead of the rich pemmican he was never tired of
feasting on.

On 31 August they left Edmonton and headed west for
asper House. On 6 September they

halted for dinner at the bend of the river, having travelled
nine or ten miles, Frank promising us some fish, from a
trouty-looking stream hard by, as a change from the ever-
lasting pemmican.

Not that anyone was tired of pemmican. All joined in its
praises as the right food for a journey, and wondered why
the Government had never used it in war time . . . As an army
marches on its stomach, condensed food is an important
object for the commissariat to consider, especially when,
as in the case of the British Army, long expeditions are
frequently necessary.

Pemmican is good and palatable uncooked and cooked . . .

It has numerous other recommendations for campaign diet.
It keeps sound for twenty or thirty years, is wholesome and
strengthening, portable, and needs no medicine to correct a
tri-daily use of it.

In case anyone should think that these references are too
old to be applicable today, I should like to introduce a bit of
personal testimony here.

While writing the first edition of this book I lived on a
high-fat, high-protein diet for three weeks, eating as little
carbohydrate as possible. I should add that I did not sit in
front of a typewriter all the time, but ran my practice and
worked in the garden whenever I could because it was spring
and a lot of planting had to be done.

I took no bread, no biscuits, no sugar, nothing between
meals except a few nuts or a bit of cheese. On this diet, which
I enjoyed eating and which never left me feeling hungry, I
lost 3 lb. in three weeks, dropping from 11 stone 10 lb. in my
clothes to 11 stone 7 lb. I was not trying to slim, only to see
if I could live comfortably on it and stay fit. I am 5 feet
8 inches tall and, though not obese, I *am* a Fatten-Easily and
have, in the past, been up to 13 stone and felt uncomfortable
at that weight.

I paid no attention to calories and ate as much as I felt
like of the low-carbohydrate foods allowed. I also drank as
much water or dry wine as I wanted. I felt well all the time
and got through my work without undue effort.

I now stick to a low-carbohydrate diet of this kind from
choice, because it gives me more energy than an ordinary
high-starch diet, and because I like it.

There was no suggestion from any of the anti-starch and
sugar doctors whose clinical evidence I gave in Chapter 3,
that they or their thousands of patients found a high-
fat diet nauseating. So it is surprising how many slimming
pundits subscribe to the view that high-fat diets are unpalatable. It must be because they have never actually eaten

them. Dr John Clyde, who approves of high-fat diets otherwise, says in his 'Family Doctor' booklet *Slim Safely*: 'Even
with the same number of calories, the high-fat diet results
in more and easier weight loss than the high-carbohydrate
diet. Ideally, then, one might look for a diet containing mostly
protein and fat and almost no carbohydrate. *But in fact such
a diet is so very different from our normal pattern of eating
that I doubt whether anyone would manage to stick to it for
more than a few days – which is not long enough.*' (My italics.)

Dr John Clyde is a pseudonym for Professor John Yudkin,
who should know better. But as he wrote it some years ago,
he may have changed his mind now.

He is not supported by Professor Kekwick, who used high-
fat diets for weight reduction in his patients from 1952 until
his retirement a few years ago. He kindly allowed me to
quote the following case which was under his care in the
Medical Unit at the Middlesex Hospital. This man was
46 years of age on admission in 1952 weighing 20 stone 12 lb.
with a height of 5 feet 6 inches. His blood pressure was high.
After a period of stabilization in the ward, he was put on a
1000 calorie low-carbohydrate diet and in a week lost 8 lb.
He was then placed on the high-fat high-calorie diet and lost
a further 4 lb. during seven days. On reducing the calorie
content of this type of diet to 1000 calories, he lost another
8 lb. in the next week. He felt very well all along and not
particularly hungry. He was sent home on this high-fat 1000
calorie diet.

In February 1953 his weight was down to 16 stone 5 lb.,
by April 1953 it was 14 stone 10 lb. and, when seen in
October 1953, he weighed 11 stone 12 lb. and felt much fitter.
His blood pressure was now normal. At this stage, he was
taken off his diet and allowed to eat *ad lib.* In August 1956
his weight had increased to 14 stone 7 lb. and his blood
pressure had risen again. He stated that he wished to go back
to the high-fat diet as he felt better on it.

The surprising thing about a high-fat diet is that it is *easy* to stick to. I have tried it myself and I am convinced of this. So are some of my patients who have lost weight on it.

Nearly all those who have been on such a diet agree that it is palatable and many, like Professor Kekwick's patient, ask to go back on it when they find themselves starting to regain weight through returning to a mixed diet containing a normal proportion of carbohydrate.

2. *High-fat diets cause ketosis and make you ill*
Ketosis is a condition in which ketones (chemicals related to acetone) appear in the blood, and in the urine.

They are produced during the oxidation of fat and are made in large quantities in the untreated diabetic who, because he is unable to deal with sugar, attempts to burn fat at a great rate and in so doing makes an excess of ketones.

They accumulate to the point where they are poisonous, and in severe diabetic ketosis, coma will supervene unless insulin is given to enable the patient to utilize sugar.

It should be explained that glucose, a simple sugar, is one of the energy coins of the body, particularly of the brain, which cannot operate without a constant supply of it. In diabetes, the body uses the other energy source available to it: fatty acids, from fat, and in so doing gets round its lack of insulin which is the hormone needed to metabolize glucose into fat and store it until wanted. But in so doing it makes a lot of ketones.

Without insulin, on a high-carbohydrate diet, the diabetic gets too much glucose circulating in his blood and it spills over into the urine which is passed in great amounts in an attempt to get the glucose away.

Before the discovery of insulin by Banting (no relation to William, the fat undertaker of Chapter 1) and Best, in Toronto in the 1920s, diabetics were treated with a non-carbohydrate diet of fat and protein which supplied fatty acids for energy from the fat and glucose for the brain from the protein. Glucose can also be made in the liver from fat, via a breakdown product called glycerol.

Progress in our understanding of the ways in which the body derives its energy and its building blocks from food has been so enormous in the last twenty years that the short account I have just given is far too simple. But from the point of view of someone trying to choose a good diet for health, the key point to grasp is that the customary division of metabolism into subsections named 'carbohydrate', 'fat' and 'protein' is artificial and misleading when the new-found insights into what really happens at cell level are taken into account.

The cells of the body operate a sort of trading market known to physiologists as the 'common metabolic pool', and from the host of chemicals in this pool, take out what they need.

Obviously, if you put rubbish into the pool, it will become choked and cease to work. The metabolic pool has evolved its enzyme cycles and responses to hormones (chemical messengers) over millions of years of dealing with a *naturally occurring* diet and that means fat meat and/or unrefined vegetable matter with its fibre or indigestible carbohydrate. On either, health can be maintained and obesity avoided. But for reasons I have explained and will return to later, free-range animal tissue is the food to which most of us are best adapted,

To return to ketosis and the people who say that it is harmful when it develops on a high-fat diet. In diabetic ketosis, the level of ketones in the blood is very high. It may reach over 300 milligrams per 100 c.c., thirty times higher than the moderate ketosis induced in the obese by fat feeding, which in turn is only half the moderate level of ketosis found in a normal person who has been fasting for two days.

Kekwick and Pawan in their studies on human subjects found that very high-fat diets were well tolerated and that ketosis was not a complication in their obese patients. Remember also what Blake Donaldson said: that in forty years of feeding a high-fat, low-carbohydrate diet to 17,000 patients, he had only struck two families 'who developed an odour of dead violets [*ketones*] on the breath when they lived on nothing but meat'. And by giving them the small amount of fruit sugar in a grapefruit, he cured their ketosis.

So there are degrees of ketosis and the effects of the severe ketosis of diabetes are quite different from the mild ketosis of a fasting person or the even milder ketosis of a person on a high-fat diet. All degrees of ketosis have one thing in common, however. They are caused by the same thing: deprivation of carbohydrate.

It is still very widely believed, by doctors as well as dieticians, that the ketosis produced by a high-fat diet is harmful, and that fats can only be utilized properly by the body in the presence of carbohydrate.

This has been expressed, in a catch phrase for medical students, as 'Fat burns only in the flame of carbohydrates.' In other words, if you eat a lot of fat you must also eat a lot of carbohydrate or you will not be able to use up the fat and will develop 'harmful' ketosis.

Dr Alan Porter in his 'Family Doctor' booklet, *Feeding the Family*, published by the BMA, says: 'Fat is burned down by the body to carbon dioxide and water, but to do this, there must be carbohydrates present. Otherwise, the breakdown is not complete and what are called ketone bodies pass into the blood and urine. This causes sweetish breath and biliousness.'

Anyone who has studied the history of diet must view this statement with scepticism. For long periods and in many places man has subsisted on an exclusive diet of meat. Before the discovery of agriculture, when all food had to be obtained from animal sources by hunting, man had to live on fat and protein alone, and in more recent times there is plenty of evidence that people remain healthy on an exclusive diet of meat with no carbohydrate except the tiny amount contained in the lean.

In pemmican, fat represents 75% to 80% of the available energy so that if fat really only burns in the flame of carbohydrate, anyone living exclusively on pemmican must be getting only 20 to 25% of the energy value out of his food. Yet this was the diet which enabled the white man to open up Western Canada and the United States.

In this connection it is interesting to note that in the backroom battles which were waged between the advocates and the opponents of pemmican as a ration for the Allied armies in the Second World War, 'fat burns only' was one of the arguments used by the 'experts' who succeeded in keeping pemmican out of the rations of our shock troops.

So much for the mythical dangers of ketosis on a high-fat diet in obesity.

What about the possible advantages of ketosis to the obese? Since the war these have become clearer and it can now be stated categorically that the benign ketosis, which develops when carbohydrates are in short supply, increases the mobilization of stored body fat for fuel, and assists weight loss in the obese.

Further than this, it is now thought that 'unless low-calorie diets are ketogenic (*have a high-fat content and give rise to ketosis*) they cannot operate by increasing the use of fat by the body but only by decreasing the formation of new fat.' I quote from Dr Alfred Pennington's address to the 11th annual New England Post-Graduate Assembly, Boston, Mass., 29 October 1952, entitled 'A Reorientation on Obesity'.

3. *High-fat diets may be all right in the cold weather, but they are too heating in hot weather*
This popular fallacy is closely related to another one: that Eskimos eat a lot of fat in order to keep warm.

Many people are surprised to learn that Eskimos spend the

time in their houses naked or almost naked, and that their outdoor clothes are so well designed that even in a temperature of minus 40° F. an Eskimo feels warmer than an Englishman in London on a January day.

To quote again from Dr Stefansson's book, *The Fat of the Land*: '. . . the clothes the Eskimos wear in the Arctic during the coldest month of the year, January or February, weigh under ten pounds, which is a good deal less than the winter equipment of the average New York businessman. These clothes are soft as velvet, and it is only a slight exaggeration to say that the wearers have to use a test to find out whether the day is cold. At minus 40° F., a Mackenzie Eskimo, or a white man dressed in their style, sits outdoors and chats almost as comfortably as one does in a thermostat-regulated room.'

So although an Eskimo lives in a very cold climate, he has contrived to make his immediate environment, both outdoors and in, as warm as the tropics and in this heat the Eskimos and Dr Stefansson, who lived with them, took a high-fat diet, composed almost exclusively of meat.

These facts about the Eskimo are not so surprising if we consider the position of fat in the diet of tropical and subtropical peoples.

The Bible is full of the praise of fat. 'And in this mountain shall the Lord of Hosts make unto all people a feast of fat things, a feast of wines in the lees, of fat things full of marrow.' The phrase, 'to live on the fat of the land', which today epitomises all that is best in food, comes from the book of Genesis XIV, 17–18: 'And Pharaoh said unto Joseph . . . take your father and your households and come unto me; and I will give you the good of the land of Egypt, and ye shall eat the fat of the land.'

Not only the ancient Hebrews, but hot-climate people in every part of the world, relish fat and regard it as the best kind of food for health. The Negroes of the American Deep South love fat pork. In central Africa the Negro gorges fat.

when he can get it, in preference to all other food. Travellers in Spain and Italy know that the food is often rich in oil, and in Puerto Rico sticks of fat 'crackling' are sold like candy-bars.

Australians in sub-tropical heat consume more meat per head than any other people of European descent except perhaps the Argentinian cowboys, who are the nearest to exclusive meat eaters in the world outside the Arctic.

Nevil Shute, in his semi-documentary novel about the Australian outback, *A Town Like Alice*, described how an English girl tried, without much success, to wean the stockmen from their three steak meals a day to a 'civilized' mixed diet.

It is clear from all this that fat is not a cold-climate food only but a much prized and essential food of people in hot countries.

To clinch the point, here is Henry Wallace Bates, friend of the great Charles Darwin, in his book, *A Naturalist on the River Amazon*: 'I had found out by this time that animal food was as much a necessary of life in this exhausting climate as it is in the North of Europe. An attempt which I made to live on vegetable food was quite a failure.'

Beside these first-hand observations, the warning cries against animal fats from the medicine men in their laboratories sound about as impressive as the twittering of bats.

4. High-fat, high-protein diets are unbalanced and cause deficiency diseases

Nothing is so dear to the heart of the dietician and the nutrition 'expert' as the concept of the balanced diet.

In every civilized country dietetics is based on tables like 'The Famous Five' and 'The Basic Seven'.

In these tables, foods are divided into categories according to the kind of basic nutriment they supply and the idea is that you must take something from each group every day to get a balanced diet and stay healthy. Yet it is obvious from what ~~has~~ been said already that men can and do remain fit indefinitely on a diet of meat alone.

Our ancestors, before they learnt to plant crops, had to subsist entirely on what meat they could kill. They survived and had children. So also do the primitive hunters of today. Eskimos who live without vegetable foods of any kind, on caribou meat, whale, seal meat and fish, do not get scurvy and are among the healthiest people in the world.

Eugene F. DuBois, MD, Professor of Physiology, Cornell University Medical College, in his introduction to another of Dr Stefansson's books, *Not by Bread Alone*, wrote in 1946: 'The text-books of nutrition are still narrow in their viewpoints. They do not seem to realize the great adaptability of the human organism and the wide extremes in diet that are compatible with health.'

Stefansson and a colleague, Dr Karsten Anderson, finally demolished the balanced-diet-for-health idea in 1928 when they entered the Dietetic Ward of Bellevue Hospital, New York, to be human guinea pigs on an exclusively meat diet and remained, under the strictest medical supervision, on this diet for twelve months.

The committee in charge of the investigation must surely be one of the best qualified ever assembled to supervise a dietetic experiment. It consisted of leaders of all the important sciences related to the problem and represented seven institutions: American Meat Institute, American Museum of Natural History, Cornell University Medical College, Harvard University, Johns Hopkins University, Russell Sage Institute of Pathology, and the University of Chicago.

The Chairman of the committee was Dr Pearl. The main research work of the experiment was directed by Dr DuBois, who was then Medical Director of the Russell Sage Institute, and who has since been Chief Physician of New York Hospital, and Professor of Physiology in the Medical College of Cornell University. Among his collaborators were Dr Walter S. McClellan, Dr Henry B. Richardson, Mr V. R. Rupp, Mr C. G. Soderstrom, Dr Henry J. Spencer, Dr Edward

Tolstoi, Dr John C. Torrey, and Mr Vincent Toscani. The clinical supervision was under the charge of Dr Lieb.

The aim of the experiment was not, as the press claimed at the time, to prove or disprove anything. It was simply to find out exactly the effects on general health of an all-meat diet. Within that general plan, it was hoped that the results would answer several controversial questions:

1. Does scurvy arise when vegetable foods are withheld?
2. Does an all-meat diet produce other deficiency diseases?
3. Is the effect on the heart, blood vessels and kidneys bad?
4. Will it encourage the growth of harmful bacteria in the gut?
5. Will it cause a deficiency of essential minerals – notably calcium?

Dr McClellan and Dr DuBois published the results of this study in the *American Journal of Biological Chemistry* in 1930 under the title, 'Prolonged meat diets with study of kidney functions and ketosis'. Here are their findings summarized for convenience with those of other doctors who reported on other aspects of the experiment:

Stefansson, who was a few pounds over-weight at the beginning, lost his excess weight in the first few weeks on the all-meat diet. His basal expenditure of energy (metabolism or general rate of food using) rose from 60·96 calories to 66·38 calories per hour during the period of the weight loss, indicating an increase of 8·9%. He continued the diet a full year, with no apparent ill effects. His blood cholesterol level at the end of the year, while he was still on the diet, was 51 mg. *lower* than it had been at the start. (Remember this when reading about the next objection: the possibility of heart disease.) It rose a little after he resumed an ordinary, mixed diet. After losing his excess weight he maintained constant weight the rest of the year, though food was taken as desired. His total intake ranged from 2000 to 3100 calories a day. He derived, by choice, about 80% of his energy needs from fat and 20% from protein. These proportions are close to those derived by a person from his own tissues during prolonged fasting. The instinctive choice of about 80% of the calories from fat seems to be based on selection by the metabolic processes of the body. It was found that with carbohydrate restricted in the diet, the appetite for fat greatly increased. The body adapted itself to a greater use of fat for energy when this substance was supplied in increased amounts.

So the answers to our five special questions listed above are all 'no'. Nothing untoward occurred and both subjects remained healthy, free from scurvy or other vitamin deficiency diseases, with normal heart and kidney function. Their bowels behaved normally except that their stools became smaller and lost their smell. Deficiency of calcium or other minerals did not develop.

So much for the 'balanced diet'. It is evidently not as important as some pundits would have us believe. In fact, many of the assumptions about diet on which national food policies are based may one day have to be revised.

5. High-fat diets cause heart disease

This is a vexed question today. There has been a steep rise in the number of deaths from coronary thrombosis (heart attacks) in the last twenty years and a tremendous amount of research has been done in an effort to establish the possible causes of this rise.

Naturally diet has come in for scrutiny and there is a school of thought, led by the American Dr Ancel Keys, which holds that a high consumption of fat leads to a high level of cholesterol in the blood and predisposes to coronary thrombosis.

Cholesterol is a fat-like substance occurring in animal fats and found all over the body. It is a constituent of all highly specialized tissues – nerves, kidney, liver, etc. It is also one of the forms in which fat is transported in the blood, attached to the serum proteins.

In coronary thrombosis it is known, from post-mortem examinations, that the coronary arteries are narrowed by the deposition of a fatty substance called atheroma. Patches of atheroma may lead to obstruction of the coronary arteries, and clotting, with death of the heart muscle from the sudden cutting off of its blood supply.

That is what happens in a heart attack and if the clot forms in a vessel feeding a large part of the heart the result is usually fatal. It is also known that in diseases associated with a high blood cholesterol, like diabetes and myxoedema, atheroma makes its appearance early and progresses rapidly.

From these facts and as a result of statistical studies arising out of them, certain correlations have emerged between blood cholesterol levels and atheromatous disease of the arteries and coronary thrombosis, *but these are only correlations* not expressions of cause and effect. It does not mean that anybody with a high blood cholesterol *must* have coronary artery disease (or vice versa), but merely that in a group of people with coronary artery disease more of them have a high blood cholesterol than in a group of healthy people.

Ancel Keys has claimed that the level of cholesterol in the blood may be lowered by giving a low-fat diet and on this basis some heart specialists have advocated drastic restriction of fats for patients with angina due to coronary artery disease.

But other workers have been less enthusiastic and Hatch and Kendall found the effect of drastic fat reduction to be highly variable. They reported in the *Journal of Clinical Investigation* in 1952 that although two-thirds of their patients with high blood pressure (and also atheroma) showed a decreased blood cholesterol on a low-fat diet, one-fifth developed an *increase* in total fats in the blood, and nearly half, an increase in the beta-lipoprotein (another fatty constituent of the blood which has been shown to have a higher correlation with atheromatous disease than blood cholesterol).

Other doctors have investigated other aspects of the problem and, of these, two of the most important groups are Bronte-Stewart and his colleagues, and O'Brien, Maclagen and Billimoria. Bronte-Stewart examined the effects on the blood cholesterol of different *kinds* of fat in the diet: the saturated (animal fats and hydrogenated vegetable fats like margarine and processed cooking fats) and the unsaturated (natural vegetable oils: olive oil, peanut oil, cotton seed oil, 'special' polyunsaturated margarines like Flora, and the various marine fish oils and animal oils).

He found that whereas a high intake of animal fat and hydrogenated vegetable fat raised the blood cholesterol, a high intake of unsaturated fats and oils had the reverse effect, resulting in a lowering of the cholesterol level in the blood.

From this work derives the doctrine that a high intake of saturated fats (the kinds which set hard when the frying pan is left to cool) is one cause of atheroma and coronary thrombosis and conversely that a diet rich in unsaturated fats (oily fats which remain fluid when they cool) protects against heart disease.

Here again we are only in the realms of speculation, for it is well known that many people live to a healthy old age on a diet rich in animal fats while others who take all their fats in the form of unsaturated vegetable and fish oils develop coronary artery disease early in middle age.

Before leaving the subject of dietary unsaturated fats, a word of warning must be given about relying exclusively on commercially-manufactured polyunsaturated margarines. They do not and cannot possibly contain all the essential, unsaturated fats that the body needs for perfect health. These can only come from natural sources – fat meat from a free-range animal or unprocessed, fat-rich seeds like sunflower seeds. To put *all* the essential unsaturated fats into a manufactured margarine would be impossibly expensive.

Attempts to relate diet to the incidence of coronary thrombosis in different countries do not support the cholesterol-furs-the-arteries hypothesis. One of the acknowledged experts in the

field of epidemiology and medical statistics has refuted the
suggestion that the intake of dietary fat has anything to do
with the rise in the number of deaths from coronary
thrombosis.

Speaking to the Manchester Medical Society on 23 January
1957, Dr J. N. Morris, Director of the Medical Research
Council's Social Medicine Research Unit in London, was
reported in *The Lancet* as saying:

What might be called the 'appeal to epidemiology' was
persistently refusing to confirm the hypothesis of a single or
simple dietary aetiology for ischaemic heart disease. In the
present climate of opinion such a negative role was exceed-
ingly uncomfortable! But it was not possible, in time series
or other series, to correlate what was known of the mortality
from coronary heart disease with what was known of trends
in fat consumption. Thus, the great variations of mortality
among Western countries having similar high-fat intake
disposed of any story that total fat consumption was the
critical factor. Changes in animal-fat consumption in the
United Kingdom during the present century could be related
to the changes in coronary atheroma found in the London
Hospital records, but they showed no relation to the Registrar-
General's figure of mortality from coronary heart disease.
The trend of consumption of butter-fat in the United Kingdom showed absolutely no relation; the steep increase in
coronary deaths since 1943 was only one illustration of this.
Changes in vegetable-fat intake followed the mortality experience more closely; and changes in hydrogenated-fat intake
were even more closely reflected in the mortality figures,
except for the social-class distribution of coronary mortality,
which did not agree with the pattern of margarine intake.
International experience was even more contradictory: Norwegians, who ate a lot of margarine, seemed to have far less
fatal coronary thrombosis than New Zealanders, who ate very
little. Perhaps the fish the Norwegians ate protected them,
but this did not seem to help Aberdeen, which registered
twice the coronary death-rate of Oslo.

Summing up the position, the *British Medical Journal*, in its leading article on 13 July 1957, said: 'Until we have more precise information on the relationship, if any, between dietary factors and coronary disease, there is no need for the middle-aged man to forgo his breakfast of eggs and bacon in favour of cereal and skim milk, followed by toast and marmalade with a scraping of butter.'

That was nearly twenty years ago and the controversy has not been resolved. A few years later, in 1962, the American Medical Association put out a statement in its weekly News Release for Friday 3 August under the headline 'AMA Council Takes Stand on Fat in the Diet'. A short quote gives the gist of it: 'A council report, appearing in the current (4 Aug. 1962) AMA Journal, is the AMA's first official statement on the controversial cholesterol question and culminates a three and one-half year study. The report was not a recommendation for the general public. It was directed exclusively to physicians as a guide to treating patients. A direct causal relationship between diet or blood fat concentrations and hardening of the arteries has not been proved.'

In fact, looking at as much of the available evidence as I have been able to digest – and there is so much published year by year that no one man could possibly keep up with it and do a job at the same time – I am still convinced, as I was when I wrote the first edition of this book in 1958, that it is refined and concentrated carbohydrate that is pushing up the coronary death rate in Western countries and not fat at all. And a lot of sensible and respected doctors and scientists agree with this view.

In March 1969, the Journal of the American Medical Association published a debate on the subject between two distinguished heart specialists. Dr William E. Connor, Professor of Medicine at the University of Iowa, argued the case for modification of dietary fat in the prevention and treatment of athero-sclerosis (hardening of the arteries). Much of his argument was based on unnatural feeding experiments with rats (what Sir Heneage Ogilvie used to call 'white mouse medicine', and not necessarily applicable to humans).

Dr Connor was opposed by Dr Peter T. Kuo, Associate Professor of Medicine at the University of Pennsylvania School of Medicine. Here is some of what he said: 'To regard an elevated serum cholesterol as a factor generally responsive to dietary fat manipulation with predictable benefits to the patient is to disregard the variability of the individual and his disease state. Indeed there are many hyperlipidaemic patients [people with a high blood fat level] in whom the elevated serum lipid [fat] levels may derive, not from excess fat intake but from endogenous synthesis [making fat in the body]. This would argue for the restriction of carbohydrate rather than fat intake.' He went on to say: 'In a group of some 300 atherosclerotic patients I have studied, none manifested the so-called fat-induced hyperlipidaemia to which we are currently paying so much attention.'

Another approach to the problem concerns the relation between fats and the clotting of blood. It is based on the observation, first reported in 1951, that, in the test tube at least, the coagulation or clotting time of blood is increased after a fatty meal.

O'Brien and his co-workers and Maclagen and Billimoria have searched for the constituent of blood responsible for this speeding up of clotting and have decided that it is a phospholipid.

(By definition, in Great Britain, not the US, a phospholipid is a type of fat which does not include the neutral fats, fatty acids or sterols. Lecithin, one of the fats occurring in egg yolk, is perhaps the best known example of this class of fat.)

O'Brien has found a marked shortening of the clotting time after a meal of two eggs, and other workers have shown that dairy products, butter, cheese and double cream, have the same effect.

How do these findings fit in with our knowledge of the

pathology of coronary thrombosis?

Plaques of atheroma are known to be present in the arteries of people who suffer from coronary artery disease. If a clot forms, blood coagulation has got to start somewhere and it seems reasonable that spontaneous clotting may be more likely to occur on the atheromatous plaques after a meal of butter and eggs, when the blood coagulation time is shortened.

It must be remembered, however, that all these experimental findings were made under artificial conditions in test tubes on the laboratory bench, not in the human body.

Nevertheless, the evidence is impressive and Dr Alfred Pennington told me, in a personal letter, that in his clinical practice he is now putting his patients with coronary artery disease on a diet which allows a lot of meat fat but prohibits eggs, milk and all milk products.

From this confusing but fascinating field of study two conclusions may fairly be drawn in respect of the advisability or otherwise of high-fat diets in obesity.

1. When a person is overweight and has already got heart disease:

There is at present no good evidence of the effect of reduction of dietary fat on the progress of established coronary artery disease.

But when it can be shown that the blood cholesterol of such patients is raised, there is a case for putting them on a dietary regime designed to bring the blood cholesterol down. This need not mean the restriction of total fat, although such a diet (which is very unpalatable) will often have the desired effect.

Natural, unprocessed vegetable oils and fish oils will also reduce the blood cholesterol, and these may be substituted for animal fats and used with a McCarrison-style diet like that given by Dr Barbara Latto on page 76.

But the most valuable single measure in prolonging the life expectancy of an obese patient with coronary artery disease is weight reduction, and if this can be achieved on a high-fat, high-protein diet the benefits will far out-weigh any possible danger from a raised blood cholesterol. The sensible thing for such a patient would therefore seem to be weight reduction by dietary means with a good intake of unsaturated fats — olive oil, sunflower seed oil, corn oil, soya bean oil, peanuts, kippers and herrings to depress the blood cholesterol.

2. When an overweight person has not got heart disease:
The beneficial effect of weight reduction in preventing the onset of coronary thrombosis is generally accepted, based on life insurance experience over many years. And if weight can be lost most easily by taking a high-fat, high-protein diet I would not advise against it.

An anecdote to end this chapter. It was told to me by Charles Best, co-discoverer of insulin, in 1959, when I visited him in Toronto. He had just returned from a conference of heart specialists who had met to discuss the dangers of animal fats in relation to heart disease.

On the first evening they all sat down to a special low-fat meal, after which they were subjected to a speech from their President on the wisdom of living on this kind of unappetizing food. Next morning, Best looked round the breakfast room in the conference hotel and saw these same doctors, all in the coronary-prone age group and many of them obese, tucking happily into a rich meal of bacon, eggs and sausages, coffee with thick cream, and lashings of toast, muffins, butter and marmalade. Physician, heal thyself!

References to Chapter 4

p. 74   McCarrison, Sir Robert (with Sinclair, Dr H. M.), *Nutrition and Health*, Faber and Faber, London, 1953.

p. 79   In addition to Surgeon Captain Cleave's book, see his article, 'The Saccharine Disease', *Nursing Times*, 15 August 1974, p. 1274.

p. 97   Lieb, Clarence, 'The effects on human beings of a twelve months' exclusive meat diet', *Journal of the American Medical Association*, 6 July 1929.

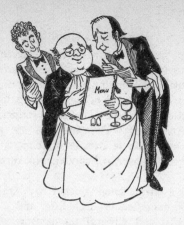

5

Eating Fat and Growing Slim
in Practice

The practical difficulties of dieting to slim are many, but the principal one is the difficulty most people have in sticking to the diet, particularly if it is low-calorie and contains carbohydrate.

The low-calorie diets advocated in newspapers and slimming magazines, and by orthodox dieticians and most general practitioners, usually allow quite a lot of carbohydrate and restrict fat, while allowing a relatively high proportion of protein. There is no doubt that people can lose weight if they stick religiously to such diets, because they are subjecting the body to slow starvation. But slow starvation is unpleasant and leaves you perpetually hungry and tempted to eat more than has been prescribed. That is why such diets seldom work for long, and why there has been an explosion of slimming clubs like Weight-Watchers, which get their results by a mixture of group pressure, brain-washing, aversion therapy, and what psychologists call positive reinforcement, which means lavish praise for any success achieved. These clubs have one other important function. They relieve the loneliness fat people usually feel, getting the new member to talk frankly, sometimes for the first time in his or her life, to a sympathetic group of fellow sufferers. The same principle applies in Alcoholics Anonymous. The members are psychologically conditioned to remain in a state of semi-starvation and to tolerate continual hunger and craving. Not surprisingly, many drop out.

Craving is a phenomenon which I have studied closely as a psychiatrist interested in alcoholism, and I am convinced that the mental and physical mechanisms which drive an alcoholic to the bottle are no different from those which drive the obese carbohydrate addict or carboholic to binges on cakes and sweets. Both are forms of addiction. (See the next chapter for development of the analogy with alcoholism.)

The most convincing evidence ever produced in support of the idea that semi-starvation results in continual craving for food, was the Minnesota experiment conducted by Ancel Keys, the father of the cholesterol scare.

Towards the end of the Second World War when British and American troops were poised to go in and liberate Europe, Keys was asked by the Allied High Command to find out what happens in starvation and how best to treat it, so that we could deal quickly and effectively with the starving millions in the occupied countries.

Keys took healthy male volunteers from among religious organizations whose members were exempt from military service and accommodated them in the rabbit-warren of rooms beneath the athletic stadium of Minnesota University. There they were subjected to exhaustive medical tests and then put on a mixed 1500-calorie diet which was a semi-starvation ration for young men required to do a full day of exercise routines and tests, as they were. They all lost weight down to skin and bone, but none of them lost their craving for food and most of them were plagued by dreams of pies, puddings and ice-cream.

The practical result of the experiment, which went on for about six months, was that the medical plans to drip-feed the concentration-camp victims with special intravenous solutions of amino-acids and glucose were abandoned in favour of straight feeding by mouth of frequent, small meals of good meat and fat with drinks of milk. Even the people nearly dead from starvation did well on this and most of them survived.

In contrast to Ancel Keys's subjects in the Minnesota Experiment, my fat patients who go on total fasts of nothing but water, some of them for months, have no hunger pangs after the first few days and do not dream of food. Neither do any of the people I have slimmed on high-fat, high-protein, very-low-carbohydrate diets. They all say they sleep better, have more energy, and never feel hungry at all.

The addictive nature of the craving felt by the Fatten-Easily who is gaining weight on refined carbohydrate is well illustrated by Mrs Brenda Smith who gave her story to *Slimming Magazine*, which made her their 'Slimmer of the Year' in their September/October 1974 number. Here is what she said: 'I'll start by confessing to a crime. My two little boys, Darren and Steve, mean the world to me – but one Easter Saturday evening, when I passed by the big chocolate eggs piled up to surprise them in the morning, I did a dreadful thing. I took the largest, carried it stealthily upstairs, locked myself in the bathroom – and ate the lot.' This little bit of thieving was not her first by any means. On Mother's Day her husband had presented her – somewhat unwisely – with a huge box of chocolates. She tried one or two and then felt driven to scoff the lot. So ashamed did she feel that she went out and bought an exactly similar box which she shared with her husband the same evening, without saying a word about her binge on the first box.

Alcoholics will have a quick snifter, a couple of doubles, in secret before a party, in case the drinks come too slowly later on. Brenda used to do exactly the same thing with refined starch: 'When friends came round for cards, I'd make a pile of sandwiches and eat a lot while I was preparing them – even slipping two or three (well, as I'm now being absolutely honest, four or five) in a kitchen cupboard as "reserves" to stuff down whenever I was there on my own during the evening.' The similarity to Ray Milland's behaviour in that classical account of alcoholism, the film *Lost Weekend*, is uncanny. Milland's alcoholic used to hide quarter bottles in overhead light fittings and other secret places all over his flat. Craving is the biggest obstacle to success in the would-be slimmer on a calorie-counting diet in which carbohydrates are allowed, or the drunkard trying to cut down his intake, without abstaining totally.

The addictive element in the obese person's compulsive eating is so important and so little understood that it is worth looking at it more closely.

Every slimming 'expert', from William Wadd with his advice to 'establish an hourly watch over the instinctive desires', down to our modern slimming magazine writers who still restrict all types of food on the same calorie-content basis, has tacitly accepted the fat person's food addiction but has never bothered to find out whether some foods are more addictive than others.

The same number of *Slimming Magazine* which carried Brenda's slimmer-of-the-year story, had this to say about meat:

It's wise to turn to the picture calorie chart which shows you that some meat dishes are very much more potentially fattening than other meat dishes . . . Did you think that meat wasn't fattening at all? Many people do. That's because they follow low-carbohydrate diets which allow them to eat as much meat as they wish, and still succeed in losing weight. The truth is that a calorie supplied by meat is just as potentially fattening as a calorie supplied by sugar or any other food.

I disagree profoundly with this statement and hope that readers who have got this far in this book will disagree too. Meat with its fat is *not* fattening however much you eat, so long as you eat it without any carbohydrate. Nor, in my experience, is meat addictive. Starches and sugars, particularly if refined and concentrated, undoubtedly are.

FOOD ALLERGIES AND ADDICTIVE EATING

Most people think a food allergy an obvious manifestation — for instance, the immediate, unpleasant physical and mental reactions which follow the ingestion of an infrequently-eaten food like oysters, or strawberries. It is not widely appreciated that common foods like bread and beer, which are eaten and drunk every day, can cause chronic, relapsing, disabling symptoms, never connected by the victim with the foods responsible, because for a time after eating them he actually feels picked-up and better than usual. This phenomenon has been called masking or the reversal of the immediate effects of sensitivity to certain foods (or drinks).

During the masking or reversal of the immediate effects, which may last two or three days, a food-allergic person can remain practically symptom-free so long as he continues to eat the food often, for then each meal containing it will buoy him up and he will only begin to feel a let-down, with symptoms like a hangover, some time later. He soon learns that these symptoms can be turned off again temporarily by a further dose of the food or drink. That way lies craving and food addiction, and it can soon lead to alcoholism when drink is involved, or to obesity when the addictants are starchy and sugary foods.

Some foods are more addictive than others. In America, wheat, corn and coffee appear to be the three foods most commonly involved. Susceptibility to wheat is usually associated with similar reactions to barley and rye. Wheat and corn sensitivity often co-exist and frequently encompass all the cereal grains, including oats, rice and sometimes cane sugar. Coffee is involved in about the same frequency and is usually taken with wheat, milk and sugar. Milk and eggs, incriminated next most frequently, are usually eaten with wheat or other cereals. Potato is sixth on the list.

These foods are either high in carbohydrate, or are usually taken with other starchy foods. They are also the most recent additions to human diet. We have not yet had sufficient time to adapt to them satisfactorily.

Finally, for the moment, it is worth noting that despite the fact that a high-carbohydrate diet has for centuries been used to fatten farm animals, physicians have been slow to accept the idea that farinaceous foods play a primary role in obesity.

In practice, the Eat-Fat-and-Grow-Slim sort of eating means a considerable change from what you may have been used to. Certain hints and tips may be helpful.

1. Try not to eat too many different things at any one meal. The more things you pile on your plate, the more likely you are to eat some carbohydrate. I have followed this diet now for many years and I seldom eat more than two or three different things at a meal.

2. Try to develop a carbohydrate alarm system, so that whenever you are confronted with a food which does or even *might* contain carbohydrate – particularly refined starch or sugar – a little bell goes off in your head and you avoid the temptation to eat it. (See Appendix B for tables of foods and their contents.)

3. Avoid what the Americans call 'junk' foods. In England they are called 'convenience' foods and include all those beautifully packaged, made-up dishes which you pop into the oven and in twenty minutes have a steaming pizza pie or Cornish pasty. Such foods invariably contain refined carbohydrate and a host of synthetic chemicals – foreign to your body – put in to ensure a meaty flavour, rich colour and

a lovely puff-up of the pastry, making use of air to bulk up the portion. A lot of air is sold in packaged foods, and corn-flakes have been described as a great way to make air stand up.

4. Only eat when you are hungry and stop as soon as you feel full. If you are off-colour with a cold or a bout of 'flu, take the opportunity to fast until your appetite comes back. This will give you a bonus in added weight loss.

5. If you can possibly afford it, get a deep-freeze and stock it with non-carbohydrate foods whenever they are cheap.

6. If you have a garden, make use of it to the full to raise lettuce, tomatoes and other low-carbohydrate vegetables. If you have the space, keep chickens and eat them and their eggs. If you like alcohol, make your own dry wine or apple ale. If you have no garden, put your name down with your local Council for an allotment. A lot of the old war-time allotments are opening up again in these days of food shortages and inflated prices in the shops.

On a diet of unlimited fat and protein with only carbo-hydrate forbidden, craving does not occur. You feel satisfied after every meal and after the first four or five days without starches and sugars they will begin to lose their addictive appeal.

Here is the simple diet sheet which I give to patients trying to lose weight. The amount eaten is left to the natural appetite, calorie-counters are thrown away and the patient told to eat the fat and protein in the palatable proportion of one part fat to three parts lean on the fork as it enters the mouth.

STONE AGE, OR PRE-CEREAL, DIET

STOP! NEVER *eat these!!*

Arrowroot, pearl barley, biscuits, bread, cornflour, breakfast cereals, crispbreads, flour, macaroni and other pasta, pud-dings, pies, sago, semolina, tapioca, cakes and buns of all kinds. And rice: a small serving of boiled rice may be eaten with appropriate dishes instead of potatoes, but rice puddings are definitely *out*.

Dried fruits such as prunes and figs.

Canned fruits in heavy syrup. Fruit squashes and fizzy soft drinks.

Sugar, chocolate and confectionery of all kinds.

Jam, honey and marmalade (except those sweetened with saccharine).

Ice-cream, malted milk and other bedtime drinks.

Soups and sauces thickened with flour.

CAUTION: *Only one* SMALL *helping a day . . .*
if you must, but best avoid most days

Root vegetables, such as parsnips, potatoes, beetroot, swedes.

Dried vegetables such as peas, beans, lentils, broad beans.

Bananas, peanuts, chestnuts, apples.

Sausages, except those which have no bread or cereal content (continental sausages like salami).

GO! *Eat as much as you like . . .*

Meat of all kinds, including offal, bacon, ham, and pork. Kidneys and liver are good.

Poultry and game, including hare, venison and rabbit.

Fish of all kinds, especially the 'fat fish' like herring, salmon, mackerel and sardines.

Vegetables of all kinds (except those listed for caution). Salads are specially good.

Dairy produce, including cheese and especially cream cheeses, butter, single and double cream. Milk (not more than ½ pint daily). Eggs.

Fats and oils, the fat of meat, lard, dripping, olive oil and sunflower oil. Unsaturated margarines.

A lot of people cry out in anguish when they see this diet sheet and ask what they are going to put the cheese and salami and butter on if they're not allowed bread or biscuits. A little imagination is required and a willingness to change the eating habits of a lifetime.

Slices of beef, ham or salami can be put between thin slices of cheese, with lettuce leaves, or slices of onion or tomato, added for flavour. And you have to get used to eating everything with a knife and fork instead of putting things on bread or toast and conveying them to your mouth by hand. Soft cheese can be packed into the hollow on the side of a celery stalk or piled on slices of apple. Meat slices can be rolled round carrots or cooked stick beans, or allowed to go cold. Other ideas will occur to the ingenious reader.

Here to end this section, and before going on to consider the McCarrison/High-fibre type of eating for weight reduction (p. 123), is a reminder of what you are going to try to do, with further practical hints, and some actual menus.

Before starting on the diet it is essential to understand clearly what you are trying to do.

1. As far as possible, you are going to avoid all foods containing starch and sugar (carbohydrate).
2. You are going to obtain your nourishment mainly from fat and protein foods, in the rough proportion of one part fat to three parts protein by weight. *This is the proportion which gives the best weight loss and there is no advantage in further increasing your fat intake at the expense of protein. Both are essential to health.*
3. You are going to let your appetite decide how much you should eat and you are going to drink as much water as you like.
4. You are not going to take much added salt, because salt encourages water-retention.

If you have a fair amount of money to spend on food this diet is simple. All you need to do is to eat practically an all-meat diet with the fat left on, with salads, cheeses and fruits as second courses or side dishes.

Although extra salt is discouraged, many other things may be used for seasoning: black pepper, cayenne, horseradish, paprika, celery seed, lemon, mint, chives, chopped parsley, mixed herbs.

Coffee without sugar, black or with cream or a little milk, tea with lemon or a dash of milk, or water, with or without unsweetened lemon juice, may be drunk in any quantity at every meal. Alcohol, if desired, should be taken only in 'dry' sugar-free drinks.

It is when you try to make the diet cost less that it becomes more difficult. Nevertheless, with the help of the FOOD COMPOSITION TABLES in Appendix B (p. 195), and the MENUS in Appendix C (p. 201), it is quite possible to obtain an Eat-Fat-Grow-Slim diet at a cost not far above your present expenditure on food.

The tables are of two kinds:

1. *Non-carbohydrate foods* (meats, fish and certain dairy products) which may be taken freely, but in which you should watch the proportion of protein to fat so as not to depart too much from the ideal, three of protein to one of fat, which gets weight off best.
2. *Low-carbohydrate foods* (vegetables and fruit) which contain protein but no fat. An exception in this table are the nuts which contain a lot of fat as well as a fair amount of protein and a little carbohydrate.

This is how to use the tables:
The meats and fish are marked to show the protein to fat ratio at a glance.

      *** means *very high fat, about ten times as much fat as protein*
       ** means *more fat than protein*
        * means *about equal proportions with protein sometimes higher*
unmarked means *substantially more protein than fat*

The vegetables and fruits are marked to show the protein to carbohydrate ratio (they do not contain fat, except the nuts which may be eaten in moderation, apart from chestnuts which contain a lot of carbohydrate).

The 'daggered' items in this table have the least carbohydrate and may therefore be taken most often; three times a day if you wish.

The items with crosses contain quite a lot of carbohydrate and should be restricted to one small serving a day. The items marked with circles are in between and should be eaten only in moderation not more than twice a day.

Now supposing you find you have taken a crossed (high) carbohydrate item and a meat dish with a low proportion of fat, at one meal. At the next meal you should choose a three- or two-star item from the meat and dairy list and a 'daggered' item from the fruit and vegetables, i.e. one low in carbohydrate.

In this way, you will be keeping up the proportion of fat in your diet which should not be allowed to fall below the ideal one of fat to three of protein by weight. And you will be helping to keep your carbohydrate below 2 oz. a day.

A little practice with the tables will soon give you the idea. Eventually, you will know them by heart and will be able to leave the book at home.

DETAILS OF THE DIET

Eggs, fish, meat and poultry are the stand-bys. You can eat as much as you like of these, preferably fried in plenty of fat, BUT WITH NO FLOUR, BATTER OR BREADCRUMBS.

Cheese comes next. You can have all you want – especially the high-fat kinds like Brie, Gruyère and Camembert. Ordinary English or New Zealand Cheddar is excellent, cheap and contains no carbohydrate at all.

Your drinks must be sugar-free. *Beer, which contains a lot of carbohydrate, is strictly forbidden.* You can drink unlimited coffee or tea with restriction of milk as mentioned above, or water. Wine may be taken but it must be dry (i.e.

without much sugar). This means claret, Chablis, or a dry white Bordeaux. The question of alcohol is still under investigation, but as Banting managed to lose weight on a quite considerable consumption of alcohol, it seems probable that sugar-free alcoholic drinks like gin are not fattening when taken with a high-fat diet.

'Diabetic' preparations will help you when you are entertaining people who normally eat sweet things. They will also help you to taper off your desire for sugar. But please do not imagine that you can gorge these things. They do contain a certain amount of carbohydrate, and should be taken in the greatest moderation. The packet, can or bottle usually states the carbohydrate equivalent. So you can allow yourself a little relaxation from time to time, and know where you are, from a carbohydrate point of view.

LESS EXPENSIVE DIET FOR EATING AT HOME

Breakfast: Kippers
Bloaters
Fried eggs
Bacon (cheaper streaky cuts)
Haddock stewed in milk
Tea with top of the milk
Butter or margarine in plenty, especially the newer, soft margarines, rich in polyunsaturated fats and oils
Midday meal: Corned beef
Braised beef stew and vegetable (no thickening)
Mince made into hamburgers
Ham (sold by weight, sliced)
Pig's head brawn, home-made or bought
Salted pig's head
Fried sprats
Boiled skate

	Sardines or pilchards in oil
	Salad or green vegetable
	Cheese
	Tea with top milk
High tea:	'Flank'
	'Breast of mutton'
	Omelette or fried eggs and bacon
	Fried liver. Vegetable. Salad. Potato crisps (one packet)
	Cheese (with butter or margarine if wanted)
	Fruit – apples, oranges, nuts. *No bananas*
	Tea with top milk
Nightcap:	Cup of hot Oxo or Bovril or Marmite
	Cheese. Hard-boiled eggs

Be very careful to avoid crispbreads, which are only breads with the water dried out of them and just as fattening as ordinary bread.

EATING AWAY FROM HOME AT THE CAFETERIA

Before you start queueing up, read the dishes listed on the big menus displayed round the walls and hung above the self-service counters.

You will be able to pick out the high-fat, high-protein, low-carbohydrate dishes quite easily.

Here is a selection of permissible dishes, made at a cafeteria in the suburbs of London:

> Egg Salad
> Ham and Salad
> Hard-boiled egg
> Margarine
> Butter
> Liver and Bacon
> Cheese
> Tea
> Coffee

At such a place, it is possible to have a satisfying Eat-Fat-Grow-Slim meal:

>Ham and Salad
>Hard-boiled egg
>Cheese
>2 pats margarine
>   (to spread on the cheese)
>Tea

FOR THOSE WHO PREFER TO TAKE A PACKED MIDDAY MEAL, HERE ARE SOME SUGGESTIONS

Cold meat (if there is some going at home) and salad
Sandwiches made of a slice of ham or bacon or fresh apple
    rings between cheese slices
Large wedge of Cheddar cheese and two apples or oranges
Hard-boiled eggs and tomatoes
Corned beef slices between lettuce leaves
Thermos of tea with a little top milk. No sugar

Suit the amount you eat to your appetite which in turn will be dictated partly by habit, partly by the amount of work you do. Remember you can eat as much as you like of the foods allowed, but if you take starch or sugar, you will stop the diet from helping you to burn up your excessive fat stores.

IF YOU CAN AFFORD A LITTLE MORE

Breakfast: Fresh orange juice, or half grapefruit
             Fried eggs and bacon
             Omelette. Ham. Kidneys. Liver
             Scrambled eggs made with plenty of butter
             Coffee and cream. No sugar
             Tea and a little top milk
             Saccharine to taste

Midday meal: Vegetable broth made with meat stock (un-thickened)

Beef stew with vegetables in it (no flour).

4 to 6 oz. any meat with fat. Mince.

Corned beef. Tongue

Tuna fish. Sardines in oil. Tinned salmon

Whelks or winkles

Jellied eels. Any fish (fried without batter)

Head of lettuce with tomatoes

Vinegar/olive oil dressing. Black pepper for seasoning

Serving of peas or french beans with butter

Fresh fruit, e.g. raspberries or blackberries in season, with cream

Tea: Cheese. Nuts. Apple. Yoghourt

Tea with top milk

Evening meal: Plate of clear soup

½ lb. meat plus fat: lamb, beef, bacon, ham, pork, veal

Tomatoes, lettuce, cauliflower, cabbage, peas, carrots, head of braised celery. One packet potato crisps

Grated cheese and salad

Tea or coffee with top milk or cream

Cheeses and apple

Nightcap: Cup of hot Oxo or Marmite

EATING AT THE PUB

Many people do business in pubs and as they are still among the most congenial eating-houses in Britain, it would be a pity not to mention how the diet may be followed in these places.

You can eat in a pub in two ways: at the snack bar or sitting at a table where a set meal is served.

At the snack bar, Eating-Fat-and-Growing-Slim is easy.

There are always hard-boiled eggs, salads and cheeses, and in the bigger places huge joints of beef and hams, not to mention fish dishes: smoked mackerel, salmon, mussels and so on.

At the tables it is not quite so easy. The set lunch nearly always includes boiled potatoes and a pudding. But usually it is possible to get a steak or a ham salad and cheese.

Beer should be rigorously avoided, and all sweetened drinks, alcoholic or not, should be avoided too.

Settle for a tomato juice, a glass of dry wine or a pink gin if you wish to be sociable and yet not spoil the effect of your diet.

MORE EXPENSIVE EATING

I do not propose to go into details of the diet for people with money. Anyone who has seen executives tucking into an 'expense account' lunch knows that there is no difficulty at all about getting the right foods in the type of restaurant that has a head waiter or in the type of home from which the patrons of such eating-places mainly come.

Instead I would like to quote Elizabeth Woody, who described a high-fat, high-protein diet for slimming in 1950 in the American publication, *Holiday Magazine*: 'A problem nobody had was learning to like meat! That's the one thing we have to thank, more than any other, for the fact that people stayed on the diet and liked it. Or maybe I'd do better to put that the other way round. Our dieters liked this all-the-meat-you-want pattern for losing weight so much that they stuck to the programme in spite of the few other things about it they didn't like quite so well.

'High-protein (and high-fat), then, was not the whole secret of the diet's success. High pleasure in the eating was apparently, the top trump. People welcomed a reducing diet that allowed them all they wanted of the food they liked so well, meat.'

For those who can afford it, Eating-Fat-and-Growing-Slim boils down to taking a diet which is the essence of good eating: sizzling lamb chops with cool fresh fruit to follow; steaks fried or grilled with onions; roast pork and apple sauce (made without sugar); mixed grills of steak, kidneys, liver, bacon, eggs and tomatoes; green salads and all the cheeses you want from the enormous variety now available: Camembert, double Gloucester, Port Salut, Gorgonzola, Wensleydale and so on.

Perhaps if we could sort out our international differences and stop spending so much money on the means of destruction, we could solve the problem of how to provide enough of these wonderful foods for everyone at a reasonable price. Obesity would then melt away and the world might return to the Garden of Eden before the serpent tempted Eve to eat carbohydrate – even the small amount in an apple.

NOTE: For those who would like to see suggestions for menus for a whole week, the Eat-Fat-Grow-Slim diet is presented in this way in Appendix C at the end of the book.

GUIDE TO THE PREVENTION OF OBESITY
BASED ON THE PRINCIPLES OF
SIR ROBERT McCARRISON, CIE, MD, DSC., FRCP

Man is dependent on the earth and its natural products for his evolution, nutrition, growth and health.

In a lecture delivered before the Royal Society of Arts in 1936, McCarrison said: 'Optimum health can be attained when – but only when – the animal organism is adequately nourished. Further, it is possible to produce at will in animals under experimental conditions every grade of health – good, bad or indifferent – by alterations in the composition of their diets . . . I know of nothing so potent in maintaining good health in laboratory animals as perfectly constituted food; I know of nothing so potent in producing ill health as

improperly constituted food. This too is the experience of
stockbreeders. Is man an exception to a rule so universally
applicable to the higher animals? It seems most unlikely that
he can be . . . it may therefore be taken as a law of life,
infringement of which will surely bring its own penalties, that
the greatest single factor in the acquisition and maintenance
of good health is perfectly constituted food.'

By 'perfectly constituted food', McCarrison meant whole,
unadulterated food, grown on good soil and eaten fresh. And
he gave as example the diet of the hillmen of Northern India
who are among the healthiest and toughest people in the world
and who are never obese on their native food. Mainly they
are wheat eaters, though they may make use of certain other
whole cereal grains.

The biological value of the proteins in whole wheat is high
and it is eaten whole, after being freshly ground into a coarse
flour and made into flat cakes called chapattis. Thus the flour
preserves all the good nutrients put into it by nature, particularly its proteins, vitamins, minerals and vegetable fats.

The second most important ingredient of the hillmen's diet
is milk and milk products (clarified butter, curds and buttermilk). The third is dhal, a pulse like lentils, and the fourth,
vegetables and fruit. Some eat a little meat, others, such as
the Pathans, eat a lot. So here is a diet of the cheapest kind
which McCarrison showed could maintain robust health and
prevent obesity. Such a diet can, with a little trouble but at
low cost, be followed in Britain today. Here are the rules:

(1) Avoid eating white flour or sugar of any kind. They
are too concentrated for the body to deal with adequately
without making excess fat, and they are absorbed into the
body too fast.

(2) Eat nothing that has been canned, processed, or
adulterated with chemicals during its manufacture.

(3) Do not eat unless you are hungry . . . and this may
even involve you in the risk of seeming rude to someone well-
meaning who is entertaining you to a meal. With practice, a

combination of tact and frankness will get you by.

(4) Eat only whole foods, from a farm that does not alter the vitamin and mineral content of its crops through high-level use of chemical fertilizers and pesticides. You may be lucky and live near a farm which uses organic methods and will sell you whole food direct. Or you may have some ground where you can grow whole foods yourself. If not, you may be dependent on the local health food shop which may not sell everything whole. In fact a number of the products these shops sell are as refined and adulterated as anything on a supermarket shelf (and often more expensive). So do not be conned. Many of these health shops are run by dedicated whole-fooders who will give you the true pedigree of everything they sell and will quietly tell you, if they think you can be trusted to keep the information to yourself, which of the foods are whole and which not.

There are also firms, run by honest people, which market genuine whole foods by post. One such is Marigold Foods Ltd. Address: 29 Bell Street, London NW1 5BY, telephone 01-402 8474/5. Cables: Calendula London NW1. They will send you their price list and leaflets and I know from personal experience that they can be trusted.

The High-Fibre Aspect of Whole Food

One of the commonest complaints – commoner even than obesity – of people eating a modern, urbanized diet based on refined and processed starches and sugars, is constipation or slow transit of the bowel contents. Witness the massive sales of laxatives of many kinds in your local chemist's shop.

So used are some people to taking laxatives that they take a ritual dose of cascara or senna every day of their lives in spite of the warnings which have been given for many years by certain doctors that this is a bad habit and likely to lead to serious trouble. I can remember Dr Charles Hill, when he was the Radio Doctor, long before television came in, giving solemn warnings against this 'repeated flogging of the lower bowel' with purgatives. Today, most enlightened doctors are convinced by the careful research work of Denis Burkitt and others, that constipation is a direct result of the removal of the indigestible carbohydrate or fibre from the diet of Western man by modern methods of food manufacture.

Denis Parsons Burkitt, FRCS, is a distinguished surgeon on the external advisory staff of the Medical Research Council, who spent much of his life in Africa searching for bowel diseases like those which afflict us in the West, among the native Africans living on their natural whole-food diets based on unrefined cereal grains and root vegetables. He found practically none. No constipation, no appendicitis, no colitis, no diverticulitis and no cancer of the colon, now the second commonest form of cancer in Britain and America after cancer of the lung. He also found no obesity except among those Africans who had moved into the town to find work and had adopted the white man's way of eating.

In the 12 December 1970 number of *The Lancet*, Mr Burkitt published a paper, 'Relationship as a clue to Causation', in which he pointed out that the removal of indigestible fibre in the processing of white flour and sugar, results in a low-residue diet and an increased consumption of refined carbohydrate. He related the increased consumption of these refined and artificially concentrated foods in England since the late nineteenth century to the concurrent increase in obesity, diabetes, appendicitis, diverticulitis and constipation, and he also pointed out that 'refined carbohydrate is believed to alter the bacterial flora of the faeces' so that they produce injurious substances which, because of the slow transit time, have time to act upon the lining of the large bowel, causing benign and malignant tumours.

He developed this thesis still further in a later paper in the *British Medical Journal* (22 May 1971), written jointly with another surgeon, Neil S. Painter, in which it was stated that historical and epidemiological evidence proves that diseases of the large bowel, like diverticulitis, are confined to economically developed nations eating refined carbohydrate. They warned that the medical profession had a duty to teach patients prevention: 'even if it entails issuing a warning with regard to such popular foodstuffs as white flour, both brown and white sugar, confectionery, and foods and drinks which contain unnaturally concentrated carbohydrate.'

Many physicians and surgeons, myself included, have now taken practical steps to follow Mr Burkitt's advice and I have cut down the prescription of laxatives to a minimum on one of my female psychogeriatric wards and at the same time relieved both the constipation and the faecal incontinence of the old ladies, simply by adding natural, unprocessed bran to their diet. Visitors, who remember the ward in the days before we introduced high-fibre, have remarked on the absence of the smell which used to make the place unpleasant to enter.

We are fortunate at the hospital where I work, to have our own bakery, run by a man who uses traditional methods and still produces a good, wholemeal loaf for those who want it. He has, of course, to produce white bread also, for few patients will eat his wholemeal, having had their taste degraded by propaganda in the press and on TV for white flour so fine it flows'. Although both kinds of bread are put out on the dining tables for the old ladies, not many of them will touch the wholemeal, so the nursing staff resort to the subterfuge of stirring two or three heaped teaspoonsful of natural, unprocessed bran into every plate of food served. None of the patients have any teeth, so the bran blends undetectably into the soft food, and they eat it with relish. The difference in the work load for the nurses has been most gratifying. No more endless changing of foul bed linen and clothing. They just toddle the patients off to the lavatory after each meal. Incontinence of faeces *and* constipation are a thing of the past. When I told Professor Hugh Trowell, a colleague

of Burkitt's, about this he became quite lyrical and said I
ought to publish something about it. This is my attempt to
do so.

Natural, unprocessed bran is very cheap. It can be bought
in any health food shop and in some chemists. Hospitals and
other large institutions which may wish to use a lot of it, can
purchase it in bulk direct from the flour mills. This is what
the dietician at my hospital does and she reckons it costs
about one new penny per patient per week. It looks like rather
speckly Bemax, tastes nutty on its own, but should not be
eaten dry from a spoon because it is light and powdery and
could easily be accidentally inhaled into the lungs. If taken
on its own, not mixed into the food, it should be taken *before*
meals, to help in producing a feeling of fullness on a reducing
diet, stirred into a little water or milk. It consists of the
indigestible bran or fibre from the husk of the wheat plus the
wheatgerm which contains the valuable vitamins, minerals,
fats and proteins which the millers remove when they make
wheat into white flour. It is sold as animal feed, as I have
said earlier, and pigs and other farm animals do well on it,
as do humans who eat the flesh of animals fed in this way,
because the goodness of the wheatgerm in the bran is
incorporated by the animal into its fat and muscle tissue.

Natural, unprocessed bran can be used in two ways in the
maintenance of good health. It can be added to a whole-food
diet to make such a diet even more nutritious, or it can be
added to a less good diet to make good some deficits. In some
situations, people cannot afford or cannot obtain a whole-food
diet: in poverty, in institutions where catering is done on a
mass scale from a central kitchen and in towns where only
supermarket-type food is available.

In the treatment of overweight, food fibre – the part of
food which is indigestible and unavailable for absorption into
the body – helps to reduce energy intake in several ways: it
needs more chewing and so slows down the meal, so that you
tend to eat less. Chewing increases the flow of saliva in th

mouth and gastric juice in the stomach, which distends the stomach and makes you feel full sooner. Fibre reduces the absorptive capacity of the intestine so that you take in less and so have less to metabolize and possibly turn into stored fat. The removal of indigestible fibre in the refining processes to which modern food is subjected is thus an important factor in the production of obesity in Western countries.

A word of reassurance about fibre should be added here. Many people think of it as 'roughage' – something which irritates the lining of the bowel as it goes down. Nothing could be further from the truth. It should be called 'smoothage' because it bulks up the intestinal contents and produces a voluminous, soft stool which is very easy to pass and a great comfort to patients with piles and other painful complaints at the far end of the gut. So-called low-residue diets (fibre-depleted) are now out and high-fibre diets are in for the treatment of all the common diseases of the bowel from duodenal ulcer to colitis and piles.

The basis of the McCarrison/High-Fibre diet for the prevention of obesity, is the wholemeal loaf, which is itself rich in fibre. In Appendix C, I have given recipes for the 'Grant' Loaf and the 'Grant' Bran-plus loaf, based on the recipes of that redoubtable fighter for sane food policies, Mrs Doris Grant, in her book *Your Daily Food*, Faber & Faber, 1974, which every seeker after health and slimness should read.

Obviously, if you are too fat, you should not eat too much bread of any kind while you are slimming, but once you have got down to your optimum weight, then a few slices of a home-made Grant loaf will keep you healthy and satisfied without putting weight on unless you are an extreme Fatten-Easily.

On an Eat-Fat-Grow-Slim diet you will not need extra fibre as bran, because the fat in the diet keeps the bowel moving . . . in fact you will know if you are taking too much ⲅ because it will make your bowels uncomfortably loose.

Stefansson and his Eskimo friends never suffered from constipation, and cancer of the bowel is unknown among Eskimos eating their traditional all-meat and fish diet with no carbohydrate.

This brings the Eating Fat and Growing Slim in Practice chapter to an end. I have tried to get round the expense factor in two ways: (1) by giving the cheapest possible 'Eat Fat' menus and (2), by giving the McCarrison/High-Fibre whole food alternative. The two approaches are not mutually exclusive, but for very obese people, the Eat-Fat regime will give quicker results and total fasting will get weight off quickest of all. In all cases, whatever method you decide to embark upon, I would advise a talk with your GP first and a medical check-up if he advises one. There are conditions which cause obesity which are purely medical or surgical and in your own interest it is wise to ask your family doctor to exclude these before you start to slim.

References to Chapter 5

p. 111 On food allergies and addictive eating, see Randolph, T. G., 'The descriptive features of food addiction; addictive eating and drinking', *Quarterly Journal of Studies on Alcoholism*, 1956, *17*, pp. 198–224.

p. 113 Mackarness, R., 'Stone Age Diet', *Medical World*, July 1959.

p. 123 Sir Robert McCarrison's Cantor Lectures, first published by the Royal Society of Arts in their *Journal*, were republished in book form in 1944 by Faber and Faber.

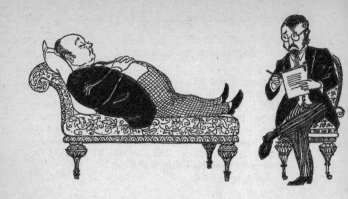

6

Psychiatric Aspects of Obesity and Food Addiction

Psychiatrists, like other doctors, come in all shapes and sizes. Some are short, fat Fatten-Easilies, others are tall, lean Constant-Weights. Freud and Jung were not fat, whereas Adler was a round, dumpy little man of endomorphic build with the cheerful, extrovert personality that so frequently goes with this body type.

Most of the popular books written by psychiatrists about obesity – and there have been quite a number – have been a bit short on psychological insight. They have concentrated on a behaviourist or aversion-therapy approach in an attempt to get the fat reader to face the realities of being overweight and to stick to a low-calorie diet by means of various learned tricks for resisting the temptation to gorge. This approach is good so far as it goes, but it assumes that there is no *metabolic* difference between fat and thin people and that gluttony is at the root of the problem.

As a psychiatrist, I am more interested in the psy

dynamics of the eating drive in fat people and the way in which, as Dr Kemp observed in Chapter 3, some people come to have 'an amazing tolerance of an unpleasant and dangerous state for what may be the best part of a lifetime before coming for treatment.'

In my *viva voce* examination for Part 2 of the Diploma in Psychological Medicine I was rather thrown by the first question put to me by one of the examiners whom I had previously ascertained was a Freudian (it is useful before an oral examination in such an indeterminate subject as psychiatry to have an idea of the school of thought to which your examiner belongs). 'Tell me, Doctor,' he said, 'what would be your diagnosis if a forty-five-year-old woman patient told you that she had gone in front of her bedroom mirror one morning and started to scream?'

I floundered about for the answer before coming up with the one he wanted – narcissism.

The poor lady had habitually suppressed in her mind's eye the mirror's evidence of the ravages of time, until one day the scales dropped and what she really saw made her scream in horror. The repressive Freudian mechanism used by such people to maintain the narcissistic fictional image in the face of all evidence to the contrary is quite common, particularly in people who were once good looking and have fattened gradually.

Shakespeare in *The Two Gentlemen of Verona* has underlined the dreadful truth which should strike at the heart of every sufferer from obesity: 'Not an eye that sees you but is a physician to comment on your malady.' Why do so many of us turn a blind eye to the truth about ourselves? Freud would say it is to preserve the integrity of the ego which we have built, supported by various complexes.

I knew a doctor once who was simply enormous. He stood 6 ft. 4 in. and weighed twenty-three stone. Bald, and baggy in eye and jowl, at the age of fifty-seven he still thought of self as God's gift to women, which he had never been even in his youth. Bottom-pinching and with a roving eye, I swear he had not had a direct view of his own genitals for twenty years.

So I suppose you could say that many fat people are unconsciously motivated for one reason or another, not to admit to themselves that they are obese. 'He is obese. I am well built.'

Stripped of all the trappings of super-ego, ego and id, Oedipus complex and penis envy, etc., what Freud said was that there is a large unconscious region of the mind which is a powerful determinant of our choices. It is sometimes easier to see how it works in other people than in ourselves.

So when there is a psychodynamic or psychopathological component in a person's overeating – and there often is – the value of psychotherapy or insight therapy, whether done in a group or individually, is to get the person (1) to see the unconscious factors which make them overeat and (2) to be more realistic and practical about the situation. Sounds a lot easier than it is in practice. Because in any psychotherapeutic relationship you get transference and counter-transference and the patient may break off the treatment before it has gone halfway. Nevertheless, it is worth a try, but no good by itself. Other factors must be evaluated at the same time and tackled in their own right. Very few fat people ever got thinner or stayed thinner with psychotherapy alone.

Obesity is very much wrapped up with the need to feel loved, and as food and love are two of our main concerns from the cradle to the grave, no wonder some people get them mixed up.

My grandmother, who was as worthy a Victorian as any of her generation, used to try to make a distinction and keep the two apart with the slightly disapproving phrase 'Like food: love people', when we children used to goggle at the chocolate cake she made so well, and say we loved it.

The food symbols of ordinary speech are clear evidence of the strong associations between food and the emo which exist for all of us.

When we say that someone makes us sick, no further explanation is required and many common endearments make use of food symbols: honey, sweetheart, sugar. Love and food cannot help being bound up together because, from the moment of birth and through infancy, we rely upon the one we love best for the food on which our lives depend.

Therefore, the biggest single psychological reason for over-eating the ever-ready starchy and sugary foods and so getting fat, is a feeling of love deprivation or insecurity.

Everyone has seen or heard of cases of girls disappointed in love who either stop eating and get very thin ('I can't have love so I won't have food either') or who start to eat to excess and get very fat ('I can't have love so I'll make up on sweets instead').

Misery is a common factor in substantial weight loss or gain in young women. Love cures both. Real, requited love that is, not just physical banging about.

This close relationship between obesity and the emotions can be seen on all sides: the mother who has no real love for her child and resents the way it curtails her freedom, who stuffs it with puddings in an unconscious attempt to make up for the love she cannot give; or the young man jilted by his girl who goes off and swills mild and bitter to drown his emotional disappointment.

Anorexia Nervosa

I have just mentioned that some unhappy girls, instead of overeating and getting fat, stop eating and become too thin. In its extreme form this condition can endanger life and is called anorexia nervosa (*an*=not, *orexia*=appetite, *nervosa*=psychological). It is worth considering here in a chapter on the psychology and psychiatry of obesity because many doctors think it is the other side of the obesity penny.

The term was originally applied by William Gull in 1874

to 'a peculiar form of disease' occurring mainly in young females, characterized by refusal to eat and extreme emaciation, which he attributed to 'a morbid mental state'. Three features must all be present for the diagnosis to be made: (1) resolute avoidance of all food which the patient regards as fattening – usually fats and carbohydrates. Self-induced vomiting or purgation is often employed after the bouts of overeating which occasionally occur during the food avoidance, which suggests that food addiction is still present, though violently reacted against. One patient I knew had to be admitted to our medical unit as an emergency, having taken sixty Senna tablets after one of these bouts of eating. She did not suffer any permanent ill-effects, but her belly blew up alarmingly.

(2) The patients have a hormonal disorder which manifests as a failure to have periods (*amenorrhoea*). They also lose their sex drive, although not invariably. I had one case where the girl became over-sexed and was quite a problem to control on the ward.

(3) A distinctive psychopathology (Gull's 'morbid mental state') is invariably present and can be identified. It manifests as an obsessive, morbid dread of getting fat. But the weight and figure to which the patient aspires is way below normal and one associated by most people with undernourishment or the stick-thin models of the fashion magazines. There thus seems to be a perceptual distortion of the body image in these people which makes them equate normal weight with horrible obesity. Not an uncommon quirk actually: many people do see themselves as fatter than they really are and will ask when they see a grossly obese person out walking: 'Am I as fat as that?' But in most people, that is as far as the distorted perception goes. The anorectic patient takes it to extremes and actually tries, in a perverse way, to starve to death. Why?

The current view is that psychological factors are most likely to be the cause and the disorder is seen as a kind of phobia or avoidance-response to the physical change puberty and their sexual and social implications. Often there is a hostile or ambivalent relationship between the patient and her mother or father.

Against this 'all in the mind' approach to causation, there are some interesting physical facts: anorectic girls are more likely to have been born heavier than average, to have had a difficult, complicated birth, infant feeding difficulties, an over-weight childhood and early onset of menstrual periods, all of which point to some physical factor; perhaps too-rapid maturation of the body at the expense of the nervous system? This physical precocity without corresponding emotional and intellectual maturation could be behind the psycho-sexual difficulties which some doctors see as the cause of the disorder.

So we are back at a possible dietary factor in *anorexia nervosa*. Could the physical precocity be due to over-concentrated feeding of fattening carbohydrates which bulk up the physical frame without at the same time nourishing the developing nervous system and brain? The final common pathway for the disorder would be the hypothalamus, an area of the brain just above and connected to the pituitary gland, which has been called the conductor of the hormone orchestra, responsible as it is for co-ordinating the action of all the hormones in the body, including those which control appetite and the menstrual cycle. Anatomically, the centres involved with feeding, menstruation and sexual behaviour are all within a millimetre or two of one another in the hypothalamus.

Treatment of the acute phase of *anorexia nervosa* has to be in hospital, with the patient in bed. At first the aim is to save life, restore nutrition and relieve acute mental disturbance, such as suicidal depression. With drugs like Largactil and cyproheptadine to restore appetite, a good nurse can usually persuade the patient to eat again so that tube feeding rarely becomes necessary. Associated depression may require ECT.

How Largactil restores appetite is a mystery, but it may be significant that other types of patient of normal weight, who are put on Largactil for years and years – as in the treatment of schizophrenia – gradually put on weight though apparently eating the same as before . . . further evidence for a physical metabolic component?

Follow-up studies in *anorexia nervosa* are not numerous, but they show a high relapse rate, varying from 20% to 65%, three to ten years after the first admission. So the standard treatment as outlined briefly above, cannot be called good. Are doctors looking at the illness from the wrong angle? Should we not stop assuming that the patient's body and mind are wrong and ask whether the food they are being given is wrong for their real needs? This could make *anorexia* a manifestation of intolerance or hypersensitivity to too-concentrated a diet of refined carbohydrate . . . exactly the view I take of the causation of obesity.

If *anorexia nervosa* can be regarded as an obsessional mental reaction against a tendency to addictive eating of starches and sugars leading to obesity – and this is a reasonable formulation in view of the evidence just set out – then what about that other great addiction afflicting Western man – alcoholism?

Alcoholism

In a paper I published in 1972 about addictive drinking I supported the idea, first mooted by Chicago allergist Dr Ted Randolph, that the alcoholic's addiction is not to alcohol itself, but to the food from which his drink is derived, like the obese 'carboholic's' craving for his refined carbohydrate. The idea goes back to 1937, when William Duncan Silkworth, MD, co-founder of Alcoholics' Anonymous, published a paper on alcoholism as a manifestation of a physical allergy. What follows on this very important question is taken from my 1972 paper on the subject.

Curiously, although millions of words have been published about the alcoholic's mental obsession, little attention has been paid to the physical allergy factor in the disease, a factor which Silkworth considered to be most important. In the dramatic words of another (anonymous) co-founder of AA, speaking of Dr Silkworth: 'From him we learned the nature of our illness: the obsession of the mind that compels us to drink and the allergy of the body that condemns us to go mad or die.'

THE NATURE OF THE ALCOHOLIC'S ALLERGIC RESPONSE

Dr Silkworth pointed out that alcoholism must be an allergy like ragweed hay fever because some people can tolerate it and others cannot. I am told that he was always careful to point out in conversation that the alcoholic's hyper-susceptibility was *in the presence* of alcohol, not *to* alcohol itself, but before he could develop the idea further he died and it was left to Randolph to apply the concept clinically.

Theron G. Randolph, MD, is a specialist in internal medicine and allergy, practising in Chicago, where he runs an ecological unit in which he works out his patients' specific allergies to individual foods and the chemical contaminants of their environment. He first had the idea that alcoholism was a manifestation of masked food allergy while taking histories from food allergy patients in the mid-1940s. Those who became ill after one or two drinks of beer or Bourbon (corn whisky) were subsequently found to be sensitive (allergic) to either wheat or corn, or to both. The point Randolph emphasized was that the alcoholic's allergy or hypersusceptibility is *not to alcohol itself but to the foods and sometimes the chemicals entering into the manufacture of alcoholic drinks.* Allergy to alcohol itself is apparently very rare.

Alcohol hastens the absorption of food, so that sensitization takes place more readily than with plain non-alcoholic versions of the same foods. Alcohol acts as a solvent for food allergens and speeds their entry into the system. In other words, addictive drinking is really food addiction, with the alcohol acting as a vehicle for the allergenic traces of the food from which the drink is made. Alcohol is one of the most efficient accelerators of the process of sensitization.

A clinical illustration, published by a colleague of mine, shows the relationship between alcoholic drink and the food from which it is derived.

Dr Guy Daynes, a paediatrician and former general practitioner in Hove, who has now gone to Africa as a medical missionary, published this case in 1959. He is one of the few British doctors who have made a study of food allergy.

After discussing personality changes which occur in some people after taking alcoholic drinks, Daynes went on to describe a case of alcoholism where wheat allergy was implicated.

'Recently I had a patient, aged 52, who showed these personality changes when drinking, but he consulted me because he was sleeping very badly, and feeling depressed, particularly in the mornings. He had the habit of drinking a very large whisky last thing at night in order to help him to sleep, irrespective of what he had previously had in the way of drink. I stopped this and replaced it with a similar sized brandy. The result was that he slept perfectly well through the night and did not wake up depressed.

'After a few nights he put himself back on to whisky because he preferred it, but found that his former insomnia returned as did the morning depression. I and many of his friends also noticed that he did not get the adverse personality change as long as he avoided drinking whisky; he just became cheerful and remained a pleasant companion.'

Daynes knew this man was allergic to wheat and suspected that the blame lay in the use of wheat in the manufacture of proprietory blended Scotch. He tried his patient on a pure malt whisky and obtained a gratifying cut back in his allergic headache, insomnia, depression and personality changes.

On first taking an alcoholic drink most people are made

pleasantly uninhibited by it. Even if they take more than is good for them they notice only mild ill-effects. This is not allergy. It is alcohol acting as a sedative drug and intoxicant, used in its time-honoured way.

There are none of the unpleasant personality changes and other symptoms associated with food allergy, which Daynes and others have described. Any after effects which may occur are far less devastating than those experienced by the food-sensitive individual eating the food to which he is allergic, or the alcoholic who has lost his tolerance to any of the common alcoholic drinks. Most people can usually go on eating and drinking without untoward reactions all their lives. Such non-allergic people are lucky because they are genetically well-endowed. Others are not so fortunate.

STAGES IN THE NATURAL HISTORY OF ADDICTIVE DRINKING

Anyone who has worked with alcoholics and taken drinking histories from them, will be familiar with the stages through which the alcoholic passes before he comes for help.

Stage One: Non-adapted

Very early on, when drinking only occasionally, the potential alcoholic will have found that each widely spaced drink is followed by an immediate unpleasant reaction, usually involving headache, nausea and depression. Such a person finds he cannot take drink as well as the majority of his companions. This stage may be so short-lived that in giving his history later the alcoholic will have forgotten all about it. In most cases it passes quickly into

Stage Two: Adapted

when he finds that if he increases the frequency and the amount of his drinking, these unpleasant effects are overcome.

This stage may be called the stage of resistance or apparent increased tolerance. Each drink is now followed by a pick-up or general increase in the sense of well-being, and if more is taken before a hangover has had time to come on, this feeling that drink agrees with him can be prolonged by taking regular doses every day. This leads to the familiar morning drinking 'to get going'.

At this point he will be particularly gratified by the respect paid by his friends to his drinking ability. The apparent increase in tolerance is the reversal of the immediate effects, or masking, of sensitivity. It is, of course, a well-recognized phenomenon in drug addiction.

The victim is now hooked, in the sense that he cannot stop drinking without a vicious hangover, and he is driven to drink often to maintain the picked-up state which he now regards as his normal form. He will feel all right once he has had a drink in the morning and can carry on drinking through the day. Troublesome hangovers will develop only after the night's abstinence. The hair of the dog relieves them. Soon the alcoholic is keeping drink in the bedroom in order to 'top up' during the night if he wakes.

Stage Two may go on for a long time merging into Stage Three in which tolerance is lost and each drink brings, instead of a pick-up, a devastating malaise.

Most alcoholics learn that they can prolong Stage Two by changing their drinking pattern in one of two ways:

(a) By resorting to a stronger version of drink of the same derivation, e.g. by switching from beer to whisky or from wine to brandy.

(b) By changing to drink of a different derivation. This is what the man in Daynes's case did. Unfortunately, alcohol is such a potent enhancer of sensitization that even if a grain-sensitive person is not sensitive to grape at first he soon will be if he drinks wine and brandy hard enough.

Stage Three: Non-adapted again

When tolerance is lost and each drink is followed by vomiting, malaise and no 'lift' at all, the alcoholic is usually also showing the damaging effects of alcohol as a poison: abnormal liver function, polyneuritis, gastritis and sometimes early dementia. His adaptive resources have run out and he is more ready to seek help.

The most dramatic case I know, illustrating the allergic factor, came to me while I was a GP. The patient was an intelligent man in his fifties, a Civil Servant and a compulsive 'bout' drinker of whisky.

He had suffered all his life from the most intractable nasal stuffiness, which was accentuated in the hangover stage after his drinking bouts. Suspecting that he might have a masked wheat-sensitivity, I persuaded him to give up all foods of cereal origin for ten days during a period of abstinence from alcohol, and was pleased to note an improvement in his nasal airway after three to four days.

On the tenth day of cereal avoidance I persuaded him to eat eight large slices of white buttered toast (of which he was fond) while I watched his reactions. In a few minutes his face became flushed and his pulse went up to over 100. His nasal stuffiness returned, and when he attempted to walk fifteen minutes after his meal, he staggered as though intoxicated. I had made him drunk on bread and butter! Most interesting of all, he told me that his craving for whisky had suddenly returned and he felt he must have a drink at once. With difficulty I persuaded him against this and put him to bed under heavy sedation. Next morning, apart from a feeling of hangover and some residual nasal stuffiness, he felt none the worse for his experience.

THE PHENOMENON OF CRAVING

Craving is one of the things which distinguish the alcoholic from the social drinker and it is a key phenomenon in all types of addiction. It is present in the drug addict taking methedrine, in the compulsive smoker, in the food addict or 'carboholic' going after cakes and sweets, and also in the petrochemical addict who sniffs petrol, plastic glue or anaesthetic ether. In each case I believe that the basis of craving is hypersensitivity or altered reaction to the addictant involved, which triggers off a physical 'need' for the drug, food or chemical and manifests as Silkworth's 'obsession of the mind'.

One other case from my own practice may be given as illustration:

A 47-year-old overweight dental surgeon consulted me because of mental depression and day-long fatigue, impairing his ability to stand up to the long chairside hours in his practice. He had been in the habit of drinking ten or twelve pints of bitter throughout the day to try to keep going and had been sucking scented cachous to disguise the smell on his breath. He craved beer if he went more than a few hours without it.

I thought his fatigue might be the allergic fatigue of the food-sensitive person, and that his addictive beer drinking might be a manifestation of masked allergy to wheat or other cereal grains.

I put him on an all-meat diet of steak, lamb, pork and chicken, excluding all foods and drinks of cereal origin. Alcohol and sugar were strictly forbidden. Within three days his fatigue began to abate, and by the end of a week he had lost 3 lb. in weight and had regained his old energy and good spirits. Thereafter he found he was able to take a brandy or two at night without trouble, and he remained on his all-meat diet with some low carbohydrate vegetables and an occasional baked potato. At no time was the amount of food restricted only the kind. At my suggestion, after he had been well for some weeks, he drank two pints of beer as a test one weekend when he was off duty. This was followed quickly by a feeling of devastating fatigue: 'right in my bones' as he put it. He retired to bed and recovered slowly over the next two days.

It would be just as wrong to say that all cases of obesity are caused by allergy to certain foods, as to call all cases of alcoholism allergic, for alcoholism, like obesity, is a disease with many facets. The manic-depressive who resorts to drink only in his high phase, the inadequate psychopath who takes drink to make himself feel socially acceptable, and the French vineyard worker who drinks to excess because the wine is available and his mates all drink heavily, can none of them be regarded primarily as allergic alcoholics, although all three may develop allergy by continued exposure to one type of alcoholic beverage.

Social, cultural and psychopathological factors are obviously important but so also, I believe, is the allergic factor in many cases of alcoholic addiction.

There are dangers in taking the extreme view either way. Unfortunately, most of the psychiatric treatment of alcoholism in this country is psychologically orientated, and assumes, without much hard evidence, that there is a special sort of pre-alcoholic personality and that if only this could be pinpointed, potential alcoholics could be picked out of the community and given special treatment before they had got into real trouble. There is no evidence to support this idea. Alcoholism is not a disease of particular sorts of personality. All of us are at risk.

HYPNOSIS AND OBESITY

Before leaving the psychological and psychiatric aspects of obesity and food addiction, I want to mention hypnosis, which psychiatric treatment properly carried out by qualified doctors who have specialized in psychiatry . . . (this is intended as a warning against attending non-medical hypnotherapists).

In my own work at my hospital I am fortunate in having a colleague of great integrity, Dr Charles Trent, who specializes in hypnosis. He has taken on quite a few fat ladies for hypnotic suggestion that the diet will be kept to.

It works well, if the patient is hypnotizable (not all are), and, provided they attend for periodic reinforcement of the hypnotic suggestion that starches and sugars will be un-appetizing, they lose weight well. Personally, I prefer to use the patient's own conscious reasoning and will power when these are adequate. But when they are not, I think that a good medical hypnotist can do wonders. As indeed he can in some cases of alcohol addiction.

References to Chapter 6

p. 132 Books on psychiatric approaches to obesity:

Bruno, Dr F. J., *Think Yourself Thin*, Abelard-Schumann, 1972.

Rubin, Dr Theodore, *The Thin Book by a Formerly Fat Psychiatrist*, Heinemann, 1967.

Solomon, Dr Neil, *The Truth about Weight Control*, George, Allen and Unwin, 1973.

p. 135 Psychological aspects of anorexia nervosa:

Crisp, A. H., *Proceedings of the Royal Society of Medicine*, 1965, *58*, p. 814.

Crisp, A. H., and Stonehill, E., *British Medical Journal*, 1971, *3*, p. 149.

p. 136 Hormonal aspects of anorexia nervosa:

Kennedy, G. C., *Report on Symposium on Obesity 1963*, William R. Warner.

p. 138 Follow-up study on anorexia nervosa:

Beck, T., and Brochner-Mortensen, K., *Acta Medica Scandinavica*, 1954, *149*, p. 409.

p. 138 Silkworth, W. D., 'Alcoholism as a manifestation of allergy', *Medical Record*, 1937, *145*, p. 249.

p. 140 Daynes, W. G., 'Our Changing Personalities', *Medical Press*, 7 January 1959, pp. 12–16.

p. 141 Mackarness, R., 'The Allergic Factor in Alcoholism', *International Journal of Social Psychiatry*, 1972, Vol. 18, no. 3.

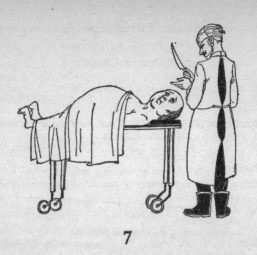

7

Other Ways of Slimming

In Chapter 4, when I was introducing the McCarrison Diet and the work of Surgeon Captain Cleave, I said that Cleave recommended a preliminary period of fasting. I shall start this chapter on other ways of slimming with the use of starvation as a treatment for obesity.

Many people use short periods of fasting to get rid of a few extra pounds put on during a holiday or in an eating binge. I have a general practitioner friend who regularly goes for one day a week without food and in that way keeps his weight normal. This is the sort of fasting that Captain Cleave was talking about when he recommended missing out meals during the day, but it is possible, if you are very fat, to lose up to half your weight by going on a prolonged fast under medical supervision on nothing but water and vitamins (and potassium supplements to prevent muscle cramps). I have been allocated a few beds in my hospital to use for very fat ladies on just such prolonged fasts.

My best result was with a woman of twenty-eight wh

a height of 5 ft. 6 in., came in weighing over twenty-four stone. She was so heavy that we could not weigh her on the ward scales (which only go up to twenty stone) and so had to weigh her on the machine down in the stores. She could not get into a telephone booth, nor could she sit down in a seat on a bus. She was acutely uncomfortable and had become so self-conscious about her size that she had ceased to go out and had become house-bound and depressed. Normally a cheerful outgoing person, she soon regained her spirits after her first week on nothing but water, during which she lost about eight pounds. She went on fasting for seven and a half months and by the end of that time had lost nine stone and had to leave the hospital because her husband and daughter needed her at home. She maintained this weight loss for about six months on the Stone-Age Diet described in Chapter 5 but gradually, because of domestic trouble, she began her nibbling at carbohydrates again and put on two stone. I was seeing her regularly as an out-patient, and re-admitted her for another period of fasting. At the time of writing, she is back to about fifteen stone, at which weight she feels fairly comfortable. But of course it is still too high.

There are certain precautions which should be taken by anybody going on a prolonged fast in order to lose weight. They should have a thorough initial medical check-up including an electro-cardiogram (ECG). This is to exclude heart trouble, which might be made worse by prolonged fasting. Provided the person is found to be healthy apart from his or her obesity, then a long fast is quite safe. Fasting for periods up to 249 days has been reported, and when I was in Los Angeles in 1963 I talked to a doctor who had treated a lady who had fasted for about this length of time.

As a method of treatment, fasting offers certain advantages over other methods: a dramatic drop in weight within one week of starting the treatment can be absolutely guaranteed, and this is a great morale-booster both to patient and doctor.

ᵗs who have tried to lose weight unsuccessfully on

various diets are encouraged to find that at last they have a method which enables them to lose. It also proves to them that they are not as lacking in will power as some of their friends may have suggested.

Contrary to popular belief, fasting is not difficult or unpleasant. After the first two or three days, when there may be light-headedness, headache, hunger pains and weakness, the stomach and the rest of the digestive tract seem to go to sleep, and although there are occasional bowel movements during the fast the patient becomes unaware of the gut for most of the time. Another bonus from fasting is that at the end of it the stomach seems to become full and satisfied with much smaller meals and in one study of seventy resistant obese patients, each remained significantly below their pre-fasting weight one year after the end of the fast.

Exercise is not restricted during fasting, and unless the patients want to lie down, they are not kept in bed. My patient who lost nine stone was very active during the whole of her fast and seemed to suffer no ill effects from this apart from a bout of muscle cramp in her legs, which responded to an increase in her potassium supplement.

In summary I would say that total fasts of from one week to ten days are a safe and effective method for anybody to use who wants to lose weight. Fasting should not be the first approach to obesity but should be considered when other methods have failed or when loss of weight is urgently required, perhaps because of the need to do a surgical operation or because the woman wants to become pregnant. Prolonged fasts running into months should only be undertaken in hospital under careful medical supervision.

EXERCISE

There are conflicting opinions about the value of exercise. Donaldson and Pennington (see Chapter 3) both used to advocate a half-hour walk before breakfast, but Cleave

Stefansson both say that exercise is of little value in the treatment of obesity. Stefansson was not a Doctor of Medicine but of Anthropology. When I visited him in December 1958 in Hanover, New Hampshire, where he and his wife, Evelyn, were running the Department of Arctic Studies at Dartmouth College, I found him to be extraordinarily spry for a man in his eighties.

Appropriately enough, my first view of him was of a stocky figure in a blue anorak with tanned face and bright blue eyes, framed in a swirling snowstorm in the doorway of the Hanover Inn. We had a meal together in the inn and I noticed that he still had all his teeth. They looked like ivory and were worn down evenly like those of an old horse. He told me that this was from using them, when crossing the Arctic, to chew through ropes and to get at the marrow in the bones of the animals on which he lived. The next day at his house over lunch, which consisted of a jug of very dry Martini and generous slices of fat meat cut from a side of sheep, which he kept in his deep freeze, we discussed the Eskimo way of eating, and also his own recent difficulty in walking upstairs because of stiffness and pain in his left knee.

He had been to his doctor about it, who diagnosed osteoarthritis and told him he must lose some weight, so he and Evelyn had decided to go back to his strict Eskimo food with elimination of all sugars and starches. Within a week to ten days, before his weight had dropped more than a pound or two, he found he was able to walk upstairs comfortably, and from that day, like Dr Lutz, he had no more pain in his knee.

We discussed the role of exercise in the treatment of overweight and he told me how, in all the many years that he had lived with the Eskimos, he had never seen a fat one. Later, after I had returned to England, Stef gave me his views on exercise in a letter:

You were bothered by my having said in one of my letters that I favoured a brisk walk before breakfast when one is on the all-meat high-fat diet. There must be some error here and I think I know wherein it lies. You had gathered, rightly, that I think highly of Pennington. What I must have said was something to the effect that we disagree on only two points that I recall: He forbids cocktails (alcoholic) and he advocates a brisk walk before breakfast; I do not forbid the cocktails nor advocate any walk before breakfast or at any other time. The Penningtons once visited us at the farm, over-night. In the morning both of them went out for a half-hour walk up and down our hills and later spoke of this as an important part of the regimen. I commented to the effect that I thought the walk specially un-needed on a high-fat diet.

Just now I am thinking-out and writing-out a statement for the symposium which results from the Conference on Nutrition in which Ev and I took part at Arden House, New York State, December 13 to 16 last. In my contribution I shall quote verbatim what I now tell you from memory. In his ethnological report on the U.S. Army polar expedition of 1881–83 the anthropologist, John Murdoch, says that he found the Eskimos heavy eaters and that the women especially keep eating all day long.

This is in accord with my observation and indeed with the comments of all those few who have known the winter life intimately. All men and a few of the women are as active in winter as in summer; but three-quarters of the women hardly ever go 500 yards from the house all winter, nor do they do any work except cooking, sewing and looking after children. And I say, as Murdoch does, that they keep eating all day.

It was in fact the non-corpulence of the women that impressed upon me the non-fattening nature of dietary fat. As you remember from my general discussions, both men and women were naked in the house all winter except for knee breeches; at Barrow he found them wearing only breech clouts. Simpson found the same at Barrow in the 1850s when he was a member of the first party of Europeans that ever wintered on the north coast of Alaska; Simpson said they tended more to spareness than corpulence; with this Murdoch agreed 20 years later, and I with Murdoch 30 years after him.

No. I never favoured exercise as such, nor walking, though I have done a lot of both.

Apart from the interesting observations about exercise or lack of it among the Eskimo women, this is good anthropological evidence that, in the absence of carbohydrate, fat is not fattening and in fact is a food to which mankind is particularly well adapted, as I pointed out in Chapter 2, on the history of diet (a subject on which Stefansson was one of the acknowledged authorities).

Any attempt to lose weight through exercise without modifying the diet is doomed to failure. Banting put the matter in a nutshell:

From my earliest years I had an inexpressible dread of corpulence, so, when I was between thirty and forty years of age, finding a tendency to it creeping upon me, I consulted an eminent surgeon, now long deceased – a kind personal friend – who recommended increased bodily exertion before my ordinary daily labours began, and thought rowing an excellent plan. I had the command of a good, heavy, safe boat, lived near the river, and adopted it for a couple of hours in the early morning. It is true I gained muscular vigour, but with it a prodigious appetite, which I was compelled to indulge, and consequently increased in weight, until my kind old friend advised me to forsake the exercise.

This does not mean that all exercise is bad for the corpulent, only that suddenly plunging into unaccustomed and strenuous exertion in an effort to 'sweat it off' is valueless as a treatment for obesity. Clearly, physical exercise must enter into the body's energy equation and it can be used in two ways in the Eat-Fat-Grow-Slim regime, to help increase metabolism and to step up the mobilization and combustion of stored fat. First, by increasing calorie expenditure. If you restrict your hours in bed to eight out of the twenty-four and do not lie about in a chair during the day, you will ensure that your muscles are active all day and using fuel. This is exercise through the maintenance of posture – much more ive in getting weight off than a game of squash or a quarter-mile sprint, either of which will throw a serious strain on your locomotor system while you are overweight and may leave you with backache or a strained foot.

Second, by helping to throw the body over to using fat. A sharp half-hour walk on an empty stomach before breakfast will make stored fat supply the energy for the exercise. If you have a dog and can bend and pick up a ball or a stick repeatedly on the walk, this will help to start your bile flowing in readiness for the digestion of the good breakfast you will eat when you get home.

Another reason for restricting the number of hours in bed is that some recent research suggests that fat people reduce their metabolism almost to zero while they sleep. Like hibernating animals, they use very little oxygen and thus conserve their calories and their weight.

Before leaving this exercise, it is worth mentioning that the many treatments advocated for obesity which involve pulleys, wheels and other bits of apparatus, often quite expensive, are not really any more useful than Donaldson's half-hour brisk walk before breakfast. The only form of special exercise which I advocate is that described in a little book by F. A. Hornibrook, *The Culture of the Abdomen*, first published in 1924 with a preface by the great Sir William Arbuthnot-Lane. The point of the exercises is to move the flab from an obese person's abdomen and to build up the torso. When weight has been lost on a satisfactory eat-fat or McCarrison-type diet, or by fasting, the abdomen is apt to be left with some slack which needs to be taken up. By following the three or four simple exercises in Hornibrook's book, as summarily described below, anybody can improve their figure and looks within a few weeks.

General rules:
   Do not exercise when tired.
   Do not hold your breath. Breathe in and out easily while exercising.

Exercise before rather than just after a meal.
Best time to exercise: soon after getting up in the morning.
Wear loose clothing.

Exercise 1   *The Hammock swing*

The idea is to swing your abdomen and its contents from
side to side. Lie flat on your back on a folded blanket with
knees bent and soles of feet on the floor, 12 inches apart, heels
close to buttocks. Place both hands, palms down, flat on the
floor beside your hips. Now you are ready to start. Raise
your hips 2 inches off the floor so that you are resting on
your head, shoulders and feet. Now swing your hips vigorously
from side to side, keeping your shoulder-blades flat on the
floor. Rest after 20 swings and repeat until you have done
60 swings with 3 rests. The whole exercise should take $1\frac{1}{2}$–2
minutes, and can be speeded up as you get better at it.

Exercise 2   *Tensing and retracting*

The purpose of this exercise is to strengthen the lower part
of the abdominal wall and restore tone to its weakest muscles.

Lie flat on the ground, facing upwards, legs straight. Place
both hands under the small of the back, palms downward.
Raise the head (chin tucked in), then raise the shoulders and
legs off the floor, keeping the knees stiff, so that the heels
come up 12 to 18 inches. The body is now balanced on the
buttocks and hands only. Move the hands about until good
balance is achieved. Try to bring your head and feet as near
to one another as possible, making a real effort, using the
power of the abdominal muscles and *not* bending your knees.
That is the first part of the exercise. Now lower the shoulders,
head and feet slowly back on to the floor and retract your
abdomen fully, trying to make it concave, at the same time
clenching your buttocks and breathing slowly out. Relax and
repeat this second part of the exercise 5 times.

Exercise 3   Pumping

Lie flat on your back with muscles relaxed. Now, gently push out the abdominal wall, making it convex (this is done by contraction of the diaphragm and will be assisted by drawing breath in). Do not depend on excessive chest action, just gentle inhalation. Then, by vigorous converse movement of the abdominal muscles, draw the tummy in as far as it will go, helping the movement with your hands if necessary. Try to get your abdominal wall to touch your backbone! Keep your shoulders and hips flat on the floor, with no heaving of the shoulders or forced movement of the ribs. Let your diaphragm do the work. Do not hold your breath during this exercise. At first it helps to inhale as you pump your abdomen outwards and to exhale as you pull it in. This is a great stimulant to the peristaltic action of the bowels, and a cure for constipation.

Exercise 4   Lateral Press

This exercise is for the muscles at the sides of the abdomen, known as the oblique and transversalis.

Stand with feet 6 to 9 inches apart, toes turned out slightly. Place hands on hips, thumbs to the rear. Bend slightly forward from the shoulders, *not* from the hips. Now retract the lower abdomen and hold it retracted, while leaning over to your left side, contracting the muscles on that side as hard as you can. To help this sideways bend, lift the left heel off the ground pressing hard down on the toes of the left foot, forcing the left hip up to meet the lower part of the left side of your rib cage. Repeat the whole procedure for the right side and do the whole exercise 20 times: 10 to the left and 10 to the right. Later, as you get better and stronger, do it 20 times each way.

These four simple exercises, which will not take you more than 10 minutes each day, will accomplish wonders for your figure within a few weeks. They are well worth combining with your diet. Keep them up until you feel guilty if --

miss doing them. Then continue doing them daily for the rest of your life.

SURGERY

In Chapter 3, one of the treatments quoted from Harvey was 'removal of exuberant fatty tissue with the scalpel'. This type of operation is still done and usually involves the removal of an apron of skin and fat from the front of the abdomen. When the apron is really big and reaching down towards the knees, cutting it neatly away can make the patient several stones lighter and much more comfortable. Some surgeons are reluctant to perform this operation because it can be long and tedious and carries with it certain possible complications: infection of the wound, haematoma (leakage and pocketing of blood in the area of the operation) and death from haemorrhage.

A more recent type of operation, also not without risk, involves removing a segment from the small intestine so that there is less area for the absorption of food. The aim of the operation is to create a malabsorption state that allows normal health but results in the desired reduction of excessive adipose tissue. Weight falls rapidly within the first few weeks after the operation and then reaches a plateau at about one year, by which time an average weight loss of 88 lb. can be expected.

The possible mortality and dangers of such operations must be measured against the poor long-term outlook for the massively obese patient who has failed to respond to all other medical measures. Although the late results of these operations are still to be evaluated, particularly the risk of eventual nutritional deficiencies and the development of liver disease, the procedure appears to have a place in the rehabilitation of these unfortunate people, who can be brought back to more useful and active life by this rather heroic form of surgery.

WATER RESTRICTION

While I was working on this book I went into my local Smiths bookshop looking for books by other authors on obesity and got into conversation with the lady at the sales desk.

She was moderately overweight and told me that her favourite and most effective means of slimming was to restrict her intake of water. Somewhat horrified, I told her that this was a most unwise method to use because she would be throwing an unnecessary load on her kidneys which would have to turn out a concentrated urine. It is true that jockeys who have to reduce rapidly to a declared weight will restrict their fluid intake before a race, but this is not to be recommended as a habit and is to be thoroughly condemned as a long-term treatment for obesity. I always tell patients that they must drink at least three pints of water or other non-carbohydrate fluid per day, and that they should always keep their urine a pale colour, never allowing it to become dark and concentrated.

But there are metabolic aspects of water retention which must now be considered. Although we now live on dry land, there was a time millions of years ago when our ancestors came out of the sea in which they had evolved as very simple animals. To survive on land they had still to carry the sea within them and this we do to this day.

Apart from the skeleton, the tissues of the body contain from 70% to 90% water. Everything that we eat has to be dissolved in water before it can be absorbed, and once absorbed it is carried in the blood – another watery solution – until it is used for energy or growth or repair by the cells of the body. These cells contain protoplasm, a semi-fluid substance, the basis of which is water.

Lack of water is much more quickly fatal to human life than lack of food and it is therefore unwise to attempt to lose weight by drastic restriction of fluid intake.

Some obese people do retain more water than they need and a reducing diet may not remove this extra water straight away. Water retention by fat people has been demonstrated experimentally by cutting cylinders of fatty tissue from obese and thin subjects and comparing the proportion of fat to water in them. Sir Adolphe Abrahams, for many years honorary medical officer to the British Olympic athletic team, discussed this point in one of his answers to a questionnaire on slimming published in the *News Chronicle* on 18 March 1956:

> One must differentiate between loss of weight and loss of fat. I have seen a man lose 9 lb. weight in running a marathon race. Of this, probably ¾ lb. was fat, the rest was water which was recovered in the ensuing forty-eight hours.
>
> Similarly it sometimes happens that, on account of the dietary alteration, the onset of slimming therapy leads to retention of water, so that no loss of *weight* occurs. After a certain time lag there is then a rapid fall.
>
> It may well happen that, disheartened by the experience in this early stage, the treatment is abandoned before the loss begins.

Sir Adolphe was here referring to orthodox, low-calorie diets.

Professor Kekwick and Dr Pawan found that loss of water increased fairly rapidly on high-fat, high-protein diets and accounted for from 30% to 50% of the weight lost by the subjects under observation.

Finally, it is worth noting that some women retain water before their monthly period and become heavier at this time. This extra water is lost when the period starts and is of no significance except that if such a woman wants to slim she would find it better to weigh herself just after a period than just before.

ALCOHOL, HORMONES, DRUGS AND STOMACH FILLERS

There is a belief in the Royal Navy, where gin is drunk pink
in the Ward Rooms, that alcohol is slimming. This is probably
true if, as in the case of some naval officers, not much else is
taken in the way of food. However, alcohol does have a calorie
value and is burnt down in the body at a constant rather slow
rate so that anybody taking a slimming diet should make
allowance for the alcohol if much is taken, and cut down
appropriately on the quantity of food, particularly concentrated carbohydrate.

Dr Pennington, who probably had more experience of high-
fat, high-protein diets in the treatment of obesity than anyone
else, said that alcohol checks the combustion of fat in the
body. On the other hand there is Banting's evidence. He took
five or six glasses of claret a day and a glass of rum or gin
most nights when he went to bed and still he lost weight, and
Dr Pawan has mentioned to me the intriguing possibility that
alcoholic drinks, by dilating the blood vessels in the skin and
making it work harder, may step up metabolism to an extent
which may more than compensate for the calories taken in as
alcohol. This increased metabolism, coupled with increased
loss of water from the skin and in the urine, could then result
in weight loss. There is some experimental evidence for this;
Professor Kekwick found that obese patients who were losing
weight quite satisfactorily on a high-fat, low-calorie diet,
continued to lose if alcohol was added in amounts up to
500 calories per day (equivalent to about one-third of a pint
of gin), but if the extra 500 calories were given as chocolate
or other carbohydrate food, they stopped losing weight and
started to gain. It is possible, therefore, that the naval officers
are right and that pink gins are slimming and I believe that
all dry alcoholic drinks (not those like beer and stout, which
contain large amounts of carbohydrates) are slimming too.
Neither Dr Lutz (Chapter 3) nor I forbid dry alcoh

drinks with high-fat diets. But it must be remembered that the stimulation of appetite and the removal of inhibitions by alcohol may mask the slimming effect by tempting you to overeat the fattening biscuits and other carbohydrate snacks which are so often provided with drinks.

Hormones

As was explained in Chapter 1, work by Professor Kekwick and Dr Pawan has shown that there is a good chance that we may soon be able to use a specific hormone which will mobilize excess stored fat from the fat organ and enable the body to burn it up. As was said, this hormone has been called Fat Mobilizing Substance (see conclusion of Chapter 1).

Hormones are complicated chemical substances manufactured from cholesterol in the ductless glands and secreted into the bloodstream to be carried round the body where they act as chemical regulators of the various organs and processes. Among other things they are concerned with enzyme systems and the control of metabolism. Lack of thyroxine from the thyroid gland in the neck leads to a condition called cretinism in childhood and myxoedema in adult life, in which there is a general slowing down of all the processes of the body and mind, and weight is gained.

Overproduction of thyroxine on the other hand has the opposite effect. In this condition (thyrotoxicosis) there is overactivity, with mental anxiety, physical agitation, and weight loss. Observation of these diseases has led to the employment of thyroid hormone for the treatment of simple obesity. Medical opinion is still divided on the result. Some doctors appear to be against the use of thyroid tablets, holding that when they are given to a person with a normal thyroid the thyroid gland just stops making that hormone and they are back where they started. But there are doctors who prescribe thyroid tablets and one of them was my old friend the late Franklin Bicknell, one time Vice-Chairman of the

Nutrition Society. In an article about the dangers of ampheta-mines (which I shall mention next) he said: 'Thyroid preparations, on the other hand, have few of the drawbacks of amphetamines and are often extremely valuable even for patients who show no definite signs of myxoedema. This is especially so if after a couple of months of dieting the loss of weight is no longer satisfactory.'

Certainly, thyroid extract or thyroxine tablets are useful if there is evidence of low thyroid activity. For example, when a person has had a bit of the thyroid removed in an operation. In such people a small dose of thyroxine (from 0·05 mg. to 0·2 mg. per day) will speed up metabolism and assist in weight loss, provided a sensible and effective type of slimming diet is being taken at the same time.

Sex hormones have also been tried in obesity, with varying results. Certainly, if there is evidence of male hormone deficiency (e.g. in eunuchoidism, where there is poor develop-ment of the male sex glands), treatment with male sex hormone (testosterone) can bring about a change to a more masculine, muscular physique and fat is lost from the feminine subcutaneous deposits. But generally speaking, sex hormones are not effective in the treatment of obesity.

Of all the ductless glands the pituitary has the best potential, and I have already described the discovery of its fat mobilizing hormone (see Chapter 1). Nature has placed this vital gland in a well-protected position, in a bony socket, the *sella turcica* (Turkish saddle) at the base of the skull, roughly at the junction of a line drawn from the bridge of the nose to the back of the head, with a line joining one ear to the other. And although only the size of a hazel nut, the pituitary gland turns out dozens of hormones which stimulate or inhibit all the other glands in the body, correlating their activities into a marvellous rhythm which, in normal health, keeps all the functions of the body running smoothly, and maintains what is called 'homeostasis', which is the medical term for harmony in the face of all the adverse things circumstances which can upset the bodily and mental status quo.

If there were a hormone to control obesity, the most likely source of such a hormone would be the pituitary gland, and in Fat Mobilizing Substance Dr Pawan and his colleagues have found such a hormone. The pharmaceutical company which first solves the problem of its extreme instability and puts it on the market in an ampoule for injection, will make a fortune in the treatment of the obese in the affluent West. Many drug companies are now working on it.

Synthetic drugs

Every general practitioner is familiar with the fat patient who comes into the surgery with the request for 'something to get my weight down, Doctor'. This request springs from the idea, fostered by our drug-based NHS, that for every ailment there is an appropriate pill and that any further responsibility in the matter can be shifted, as if by magic, from the patient to the doctor by the simple procedure of writing a prescription for the latest pill.

Drugs for obesity fall into three main classes:

(1) Aperients, purgatives and laxatives which act on the bowel;
(2) Appetite suppressants which act by taking away hunger and sometimes cause nausea (Lester Piggott, the jockey, smokes a big cigar before meals);
(3) Substances which have a specific fat-mobilizing effect on the fat stores in the fat organ.

(1) Laxatives like magnesium sulphate (Epsom salts) are among the oldest drugs used for slimming and will get weight off temporarily if they cause diarrhoea, malabsorption of food and loss of water from the bowel. But the resulting thirst will put a lot of the weight back in the form of water needed by the dehydrated body.

Continual abuse of saline purgatives can seriously interfere with the digestion and absorption of essential nutrients as well as of calorie-laden starches and sugars, and will eventually lead to lack of tone in the bowel which will cease to pass the food along. An intestinal obstruction requiring surgical treatment may be the result. One lady I knew, who took salts every day, was one day rushed off to hospital where she had to have a piece of her bowel removed because it had blown up like a balloon, under the continual stimulus of the laxatives which she took for slimming.

(2) Appetite suppressants such as amphetamine, Tenuate, Filon, etc., all act via the central nervous system and its centres for hunger and satiety. They also stimulate mental and physical activity, stepping up the output side of the energy equation. After the first burst of enthusiasm for them, they have all been found to be more or less addictive and the prescription of many of them has been curbed by Government order. Nevertheless, there is a flourishing black market in these drugs which can cause serious psychiatric problems for those who abuse them.

With the appetite-depressant drugs, it is convenient to take the low- or non-calorie stomach fillers like methyl cellulose, which act by expanding and filling up the stomach so that it thinks it has had a good meal and no longer gives hunger-pang signals which might tempt the patient to nibble.

Many of the patent biscuits and slimming packet-meals sold in chemists contain these stomach fillers so that the slimmer can get the impression that a good-sized meal is being taken. The manufacturers have taken the trouble to put in some good protein and some vitamins, so that under-nourishment is to some extent guarded against. The snag is that these patent slimming foods are expensive and may be lacking in some essential nutrients like certain unsaturated fats which the body must have ready-made to keep healthy, but which have not the shelf-life required of a patent slimming food sold in a chain store. My experience with patients trying to slim with these patent biscuits, soups and so on, is that they either do not stick to them for long enough or regard them as in some way 'slimming' irrespective of the calories they contain. 'I've had my slimming food,' they say. 'Now I am going to have lunch.'

Although amphetamines and other brain-stimulating drugs are bad and should never be used for slimming, other drugs such as the polynitrophenols, which cause wasting of the whole body, are very much worse. They are no longer readily available in Britain but can still be obtained in some countries abroad. They should be avoided like the plague, as they can induce anaemia, tuberculosis and serious ill-health, far worse than the obesity the drugs are meant to treat.

(3) Fenfluramine (Ponderax) is a new slimming drug which has been on the market, on prescription only, since 1962. Its action is different from other drugs mentioned so far, in that it has a lipolytic effect, i.e. it helps to mobilize fat from the fat stores. It also reduces lipid synthesis (stops you making more fat).

In doses from 20 to 160 mg. per day, fenfluramine induces a significant increase in free fatty acids and ketones in the plasma. In other words, like the hormone FMS, it has a fat-mobilizing action and in that sense works directly on the excess fat stores as a slimming drug. Cholesterol levels after fenfluramine are unaffected.

In case anyone should think that in this drug the answer to the slimmer's prayers has been found, I should add that not everyone can take it without feeling terrible (I am one such) and that cases of fenfluramine psychosis have been reported, which is to say that it can make some people go temporarily mad.

Still, it is a significant advance in the search for the key to obesity and the great amount of research work that its makers,

Selpharm Laboratories Ltd, have put into it, has taken our understanding of the physiology and biochemistry of the fat organ and its disorders a step further.

HIGH-PROTEIN, LOW-FAT DIETS

Most popular slimming diets in magazines and newspapers are now in this category, with or without calorie-counting. They are bad because they tend to restrict essential fats which the body and particularly the nervous system *must* have to stay healthy.

Stefansson, during the all-meat diet experiment at Bellevue Hospital, New York, already referred to (Chapter 4, p. 96), had been put on exclusively lean meat at the suggestion of Dr DuBois who was in charge. Here is what happened (from pp. 68 and 69 of Stefansson's book *The Fat of the Land*):

> The experiment started smoothly with Andersen (his explorer colleague), who was permitted to eat in such quantities as he liked, such things as he liked, provided they came under our definition of meat.
>
> In my case there was a hitch, in a way foreseen. For I had published in 1913, on pages 140–2 of *My Life with the Eskimo*, an account of how some natives and I became ill when we were forced to go two or three weeks on lean meat. So I forecast trouble when DuBois suggested that I start the test by eating as large quantities as I possibly could of chopped, fatless muscle. But he countered by citing my own experience where illness had not come until after more than a week, and he now proposed lean for only two or three days. So I gave in.
>
> The chief purpose of placing me abruptly on exclusively lean was that there would be a sharp contrast with Andersen, who was going to be on a normal meat diet, consisting of such proportions of lean and fat as his own taste determined.
>
> In the Arctic we had become ill during the second or third fatless week. I now became ill on the second day. The time difference between Bellevue and the Arctic was due no d

mainly to the existence of a little fat, here and there, in our northern caribou – we had eaten the tissue from behind the eyes, we had broken the bones for marrow, and in doing everything we could to get fat we had evidently secured more than we realized. At Bellevue the meat, carefully scrutinized, was as lean as such muscle tissue well can be. Then, in the Arctic we had eaten tendons and other indigestible matter, we had chewed the soft ends of bones, getting a deal of bulk that way when we were trying to secure fat. What we ate at Bellevue contained no bulk material of this kind, so that my stomach could be compelled to hold a much larger amount of lean. Moreover, I had in New York a much larger stomach than in the Arctic; there it had been constricted in accord with the small bulk of a lean-fat diet; here in 'civilization' it had been expanded through the needs of a bulky mixed diet.

The symptoms brought on at Bellevue by an incomplete meat diet (this ration of lean without fat) were exactly the same as in the Arctic, except that they came on faster – diarrhoea and a feeling of general baffling discomfort.

Up North the Eskimos and I had been cured immediately when we got some fat. Dr DuBois now cured me the same way, by giving me fat sirloin steaks, brains fried in bacon fat, and things of that sort. In two or three days I was all right, but I had lost considerable weight.

A second upset was a result of the first, and a result, too, of carelessness. As has been said, my cure from the lean-meat difficulty was in part the eating of brains fried in bacon fat. The brains tasted delicious, partly no doubt on their own merits but also partly on account of the bacon fat through which we were compensating for the previous excess of lean; so I ate too much. This produced a mild indigestion, with attendant discomforts, and reminded me that the only recurrent digestive upsets I had had on our exclusive meat up North were those produced by eating large meals which contained too high a percentage of fat, which was most likely to occur just after we had been living on meat that was too lean.

There is no tendency to overeat of fat if you have fat ry day (not necessarily at every meal); but there is danger of it after a shortage of fat. So far as memory serves and my records go, there is no corresponding tendency to overeat of lean to an injurious extent after one has been on an excessively fat regimen.

Two lessons for Eat-Fat-Grow-Slim slimmers can be learned from this testimony from Dr Stefansson:

(1) You cannot eat too much fat all at once without running the risk of digestive upset. So, in fact, the intake of fat limits itself.

(2) Protein alone – absolutely lean meat or fish – is not compatible with good health. It gives rise to a sense of unease and to diarrhoea. This is because fat is as necessary to life and well-being as any other vital food. Go without it completely for even a few days and you will feel ill.

Since neither Stefansson nor Karsten Andersen ate any carbohydrate during their all-meat year, obviously people can get on quite well without any carbohydrate at all.

GROUP THERAPY

An enterprising lady, Mrs Bernice Weston, has in recent years made a good thing out of group therapy for the obese in her Weight Watchers Clubs. Although some people cannot get on at all in the group situation of the Weight Watchers, and resent having to pay every time they attend, others do very well, and the success of Mrs Weston's idea is proved by the many imitators who have started groups under other names and even publish specialist magazines for slimmers.

The Weight Watcher programme involves a low-calorie diet with quite a lot of carbohydrate, and public weighing of the members at the meetings. The group pressures to conform and stick to the diet are considerable and backsliders can expect critical comments while those who do well get praise.

One good thing about Weight Watchers is that they insist on the meals all being eaten and at the proper time, th·

ensuring adequate nutrition and avoiding the folly of missing breakfast and going to work on an empty stomach, with resulting fatigue and poor work performance. It is better to fast altogether than to miss odd meals – especially breakfast, which, if taken as fat and protein, will sustain you right through the morning and ensure that you need only a light lunch.

I think Weight Watchers would get better results with either a high-fat, high-protein, low-carbohydrate or McCarrison/Cleave-type diet, and I have known members who have dropped out because the diet prescribed by Mrs Weston leaves them always hungry as low-calorie, carbohydrate-containing diets usually do.

It is not intended that all these alternative methods of slimming be adopted indiscriminately. Some are more scientifically-based than others, while some may suit one person more than another. In the next and final chapter, 'Summing Up' the whole subject of slimming will be put into perspective and I shall give my final recommendations.

References to Chapter 7

p. 148 Harden, R. M., 'Total Fasting in the Treatment of Obesity',
Medical News Magazine Symposium on Obesity, January
1967, p. 5.

p. 154 Hornibrook, F. A., *The Culture of the Abdomen*, Penguin
Books, 1957.

p. 157 Surgical operations for obesity:
Payne, J. H., and de Wind, L. T., *American Journal of
Surgery*, 1969, *118*, p. 141.

p. 166 DuBois, Eugene F., 'The Control of Protein in the Diet',
Journal of the American Dietetic Association, 1928.

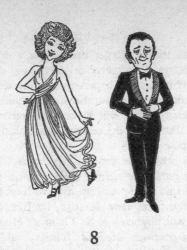

8

The Dangers and Prevention of Obesity

So far, little has been said about the dangers and disadvantages of being overweight. This is because very little needs to be said that a fat person does not know only too well already.

At the risk of depressing the overweight reader, a few figures on longevity and the incidence of disease in relation to obesity will now be given. With the means of slimming effectively and painlessly already in his hand, it is perhaps legitimate to present facts which may scare him into doing something about getting his weight down. Mr McNeill Love, surgeon to the Royal Northern Hospital in London and co-author of that 'Bible' of surgery known affectionately to generations of medical students as *Bailey and Love*, wrote in a paper on the surgical hazards of obesity: 'A well-known insurance society states that a person fifty years of age who is 50 lb. over-weight, has reduced his expectation of life by 50%. Increased risks are also reflected in the mortality and morbidity of the obese when surgical procedures are required.'

Fat people tend to forget that not only do they run an increased risk of dying early or developing diseases which interest the physician like hypertension, diabetes, arthritis and coronary thrombosis, but also that if they should ever have to have an operation they will make the surgeon swear as he struggles to distinguish the relevant anatomical landmarks in a sea of adipose tissue.

And even when the surgeon has managed to find the appendix or repair the hernia, the fat man's post-operative progress is bound to be poor compared with his lean brother's.

Next, a physician's view. In 1952, Dr John S. Richardson (then consultant physician to St Thomas's Hospital), writing in the *Post-graduate Medical Journal*, said: 'Insurance statistics show that between the ages of 45 and 50 for every 10 lb. over-weight there is roughly a 10% increase in the death-rate over the average for that age. This is largely a result of cardiovascular and renal disease' (diseases of heart, blood-vessels and kidneys).

Lastly, life insurance examination, the most ruthless estimate of our chances.

The late Dr A. Hope Gosse, TD, MD, FRCP, formerly consulting physician to St Mary's and the Brompton Hospital, writing on obesity from the point of view of the insurance medical officer in the same number of the *Post-graduate Medical Journal*: 'Both for life assurance and sickness insurance the two commonest causes of "loading" the premium are to be found in the figures for the weight or blood pressure of the proposer, when such figures are regarded as above the average for his height and age.'

These are some of the dangers of obesity and it is clear that they increase as the weight goes up beyond what it should be for height and build.

Luckily the converse is also true. As a fat person's weight comes down so his chances of developing those diseases known to be associated with obesity become less and his expectation of life increases. This was strikingly demonstrated by Dr Alfred Pennington when he slimmed the executives of du Pont, the American chemical firm, on an unrestricted calorie, high-fat, high-protein diet similar to the one advocated in this book.

Shortly after the last war, the Medical Division of du Pont became concerned about the obesity of some of the staff and gave Dr Pennington the job of finding out why orthodox low-calorie diets were so conspicuously unsuccessful in dealing with the problem. After some thorough research, Pennington came to the conclusion that Banting was right and that obesity is caused not by overeating but by an inability to utilize carbohydrate for anything except making fat.

He decided to by-pass this block in the pathway from starch and sugar to energy by withholding these foods, and gave fat and protein instead, in the proportion of one to three by weight (Stefansson's proportion on his year's all-meat diet). The results amply justified all the ground work he had put in.

Here is part of a report of an interview he gave to Elizabeth Woody, published in a supplement to the American *Holiday Magazine*:

Of the twenty men and women taking part in the test, all lost weight on a diet in which the total calorie intake was unrestricted. The basic diet totalled about 3,000 calories per day, but meat and fat in any desired amount were allowed those who wanted to eat still more. The dieters reported that they felt well, enjoyed their meals and were never hungry between meals. Many said they felt more energetic than usual; none complained of fatigue. Those who had high blood pressure to begin with were happy to be told by the doctors that a drop in blood pressure paralleled their drop in weight.

The twenty 'obese individuals', as the paper unflatteringly terms them, lost an average of twenty-two pounds each, in an average time of three and a half months. The range of weight loss was from nine to fifty-four pounds and the range of time was from about one and a half to six months.

With regard to the discomforts and disadvantages of obesity, it is appropriate to return to William Banting, whose work has had to wait a hundred years for proper recognition.

When his *Letter on Corpulence* was published, medical men called his system a humbug and held it up to ridicule. In those days of aggressive drugging and violent purgation this was to be expected.

Let him speak for himself in his delightful nineteenth-century English:

Oh! that the faculty would look deeper into and make themselves better acquainted with the crying evil of obesity – that dreadful tormenting parasite on health and comfort. Their fellow-men might not descend into early premature graves, as I believe many do, from what is termed apoplexy, and certainly would not, during their sojourn on earth, endure so much bodily and consequently mental infirmity.

Corpulence, though giving no actual pain, as it appears to me, must naturally press with undue violence upon the bodily viscera, driving one part upon another, and stopping the free action of all. I am sure it did in my particular case, and the result of my experience is briefly as follows:

I have not felt so well as now for the last twenty years. Have suffered no inconvenience whatever in the probational remedy. Am reduced many inches in bulk, and 35 lb. in weight in thirty-eight weeks. Come down stairs forward naturally, with perfect ease. Go up stairs and take ordinary exercise freely, without the slightest inconvenience. Can perform every necessary office for myself. The umbilical rupture is greatly ameliorated, and gives me no anxiety. My sight is restored – my hearing improved. My other bodily ailments are ameliorated; indeed, almost passed into matter of history.

It is still unfortunately true that many doctors do not understand obesity for what it is: a failure of adaptation to a diet based largely on refined carbohydrate; a misuse of the body evolved to deal with Stone-Age food, by feeding it concentrated fuel (calories) instead of wholesome nourishm

The standard medical approach to obesity in this country is still to give the patient a low-calorie diet sheet, with or without some pills to depress appetite, and to leave him to try and starve the fat off. Banting received the same kind of treatment before he consulted Mr Harvey. Slimming 'experts' still write this sort of stuff: 'The problem of slimming boils down to the quite simple one of reducing the total amount of food eaten . . . If you are putting on weight, you are consuming more energy in the form of food than you are expending in the form of physical exertion.' No suggestion here that excessive fat storage might be independent either of the food intake or the energy expenditure or both. Nor any mention of the possibility that different kinds of food might be metabolized differently in fat and in thin people.

Since *Eat Fat and Grow Slim* was first published, two other books by doctors, telling substantially the same story, have been widely read: Herman Taller's *Calories Don't Count*, and more recently the highly successful *Dr Atkins' Diet Revolution*. Of course neither of these two books – nor mine – is revolutionary in the true sense of that much-abused word. They state well-attested facts about obesity which have been persistently ignored by the medical profession as a whole since Banting and Harvey first put them forward over 100 years ago.

Why do the majority of doctors go on dishing out low-calorie diet sheets and ignoring the output side of the energy equation? Why do they swallow the very dubious theory that animal fats are dangerous? Several reasons. First, medical education is still, in spite of attempted reforms, among the most authoritarian and hierarchical in the world, partly because of the mass of facts that have to be crammed into the unfortunate medical student's head in a short space of time.

Secondly, because of the ladder structure of advancement in hospital medicine, the junior who questions the dogmas of his teachers and seniors is branded as a trouble-maker and

his progress to consultant status made that much more difficult. In theory, the bright, questioning lad is encouraged to
make new discoveries or at least overturn outworn practices,
but in fact he usually ends up treading on some powerful big-
wig's corns, with dire consequences for his future prospects.
It happens in other walks of life too. Aspiring young
politicians, architects or lawyers have to speak nicely to the
people above them or they are likely to come unstuck.

In my own case, although I have occasionally managed to
keep my mouth shut when a senior man is voicing some cock-
eyed opinion, I am a born agitator. I've never held a consultant post and have now, after thirty years in medicine, opted
for a pleasant assistant psychiatrist job which not only gives
me the chance to spend as much time with patients as I like
but also gives me time to write. 'Why don't you go for a
consultant post, Mac?' friends have often asked. 'God forbid,'
I now reply. And secretly, many of my consultant friends
agree with me. After struggling for years up the ladder on
low pay and long hours, they find that now they've got to
the top there are no longer the juniors to serve them as they
in their time served their old-time masters, and that the pay
and status have been devalued. No wonder the younger ones
emigrate.

Thirdly, textbooks take a long time to write and publish,
and bringing them up to date is a formidable task. So most
textbooks of medicine on which students and doctors rely
are years out of date. Here is a little gem from that epitome
of medical orthodoxy, the *Principles and Practice of Medicine*
(8th edition, 1967, p. 462 – if anyone wants to check):

Fat. A diet providing 1000 Cal. containing 100 G. of carbohydrate and 60 G. of protein, cannot include more than 40 G.
of fat. This allowance of fat, though small, is sufficient to
make the diet palatable and acceptable to the patient.
    Recently, popular books and newspaper articles have stated
that there is no need to restrict the intake of fat in obese

patients. Eat Fat and Get Slim is advice which has an obvious appeal. In clinical practice this advice is of no therapeutic value since patients could not be expected to tolerate for more than a short time a bizarre diet which is rich in fat and low in carbohydrate and one which ultimately fails to cause a greater weight loss than the properly balanced diet described above.

Finally, more perhaps than people in any other profession, doctors are conventional and hate changing their ideas. Also, in common with the rest of humanity, they are lazy and nothing is such hard work as constructive thinking. But, to be fair, there are shining exceptions to this rule and it has been my good fortune to know and work with some of them. It is really the middle-echelon consultants who are stuffy. The real big boys are not. Many are as open-minded as you could wish and one of these is Professor John McMichael, lately Director of the British Postgraduate Medical Federation in London.

For an up-to-date and balanced view on the fats and coronary thrombosis controversy, I would like to quote from a letter which he published on the subject in *The Lancet* of 29 June 1974. It was headed 'Diet and Exercise in Coronary Heart Disease' and began: 'Sir – I am at a loss to understand why some well-known colleagues are propagating by press and radio advice to the public which is likely to disturb the life habits of many people, but with such slender evidence of likely benefit.' He went on to quote from a recently issued advisory booklet from the International Society of Cardiologists (a most influential body of heart specialists) which said: an increased intake of cholesterol and fat is an absolute prerequisite for the experimental production of severe atherosclerosis (the 'furring of the arteries' which often precedes a heart attack). 'This,' wrote Professor McMichael, 'is quite unsubstantiated.'

He went on to attack the widely held idea that active physical exercise protects against heart attacks and to quote the careful follow-up studies published by the National Heart Institute, which denied any beneficial effect from exercise. He quoted from a paper by Dr Wallace Yater and others in the *American Heart Journal* (1948) which analysed 450 post-mortems on men between eighteen and thirty-nine years of age, in the US Armed Forces, who had died of heart attacks. It showed that 27% of the attacks came on during vigorous physical exercise. 'Considering the fraction of our time spent in strenuous activities,' commented McMichael, 'this is a striking demonstration that exercise can be an important precipitating factor.' He finished the letter, which was long and detailed, with nineteen references to published scientific work, saying: 'It does our profession little credit to continue basing rules for advice and management on such uncertain and highly improbable hypotheses.'

Professor McMichael is one of the most respected physicians in the world and beside his opinions, statements like those of Professor Yudkin, who works closely with the food manufacturing industry, have limited value.

Unlike Yudkin who is a physiologist and Ancel Keys the American biochemist who started the cholesterol scare, Professor McMichael has spent a lifetime in medicine actually looking after patients at one of the leading teaching hospitals in London. His views must command more respect than those of people who work in laboratories and make ex-cathedra statements which are seized upon by one or other segment of the food manufacturing industry.

What is badly needed at this stage in our struggle to control the epidemics of obesity, coronary thrombosis and degenerative disease, is some independent control of the food manufacturers and the medical and scientific people they employ.

Our food is literally our life-blood and its manufacture and marketing is far too important to the future health of our people for it to be left to profit-orientated firms like Booker McConnell, the sugar people, or Ranks the flour millers. The Government exerts ever-stricter control over the drug industry, but this is stable-door locking. The horse of national health has already bolted, sick in mind and body, knackered by the food on which we have allowed it to be reared by a free-booting food industry.

In the Ministry of Agriculture and Fisheries, we already have the nucleus of a Government organization which, expanded and with the recruitment of some non-committed scientists and doctors, could organize a supply of good, wholesome food for the people of this country which in twenty years could transform our health, cut the cost of the NHS by half and make the drug industry far less of a burden on the taxpayer.

All that is needed is to stop basing the feeding of the nation on refined sugar, white flour and chemically adulterated 'made-up' foods, and to start applying the sound principles of nutrition put forward by Stefansson, McCarrison and Cleave. Stop feeding the public useless calories and begin giving them properly constituted whole food.

This brings me to the subject of the prevention of obesity, which goes hand-in-hand with the promotion of good health in infancy and childhood.

No child ever became obese on human breast milk. It is an ideal food for human babies, uniquely designed to furnish all the baby needs for growing a healthy body and nervous system. It is unfortunate that the media have for years cultivated the image of the half-lemon, tip-tilted upwards, as the ideal form for the human female breast. Breast-feeding, as anyone who has done a lot of it will tell you, converts the mother's breast first into a bunch of grapes and eventually into a razor strop. And razor strops do not rate highly as sex symbols. Eileen Fowler, the BBC Radio exercise lady, will doubtless be able to tell any nursing mother some exercises which will restore her breasts to half-lemons or at least fairly tight bunches of grapes after breast-feeding, but in my experience, few patients persist with such exercises for long enough for them to have the desired effect. What is really required is a shift of emphasis from adolescent tit-worship to a genuine concern for what is best for babies.

And there is no doubt that breast-feeding is best for babies. Ninety-five per cent of all babies could and should be breast-fed for the first six months of life at least. Compared with any commercial milk formula, breast milk is cleaner, cheaper and nutritionally better suited to the baby's needs. It provides immunity to some infections at a time when the baby has not yet developed immunity for itself. It provides physical and face-to-face contact between mother and child, which psychologists now believe to be essential for the full emotional development of both. Several research teams have shown that there is a critical time – quite a short period of weeks – during which, if overfeeding with starches and sugars takes place, MORE THAN THE NORMAL NUMBER OF FAT CELLS WILL BE FORMED – and they will never go away, they are with the child for the rest of its life, a built-in tendency to obesity. Bottle-feeding will do this, if the formula is too sweet.

In well-off families, bottle-feeding is a means whereby the mother gains greater freedom for social and professional pursuits and also preserves her figure. She would do better to hire a wet nurse. Unfortunately, if the rich bottle-feed, the less well-off will aspire to do so also, and this aspiration is being exploited by the food manufacturers who market milk powders in under-developed countries. So serious has the situation become that the international aid agency, War on Want, published a report recently in which the baby food industry is accused of promoting its products in communities which cannot use them properly, and of using sophisticated advertising tricks – girls dressed as nurses, samples and free gifts, to persuade uneducated mothers to give up breast-feeding. Wealthy, well-educated mothers can probably get away with bottle-feeding their infants without too much risk of infection, but they run the risk of laying the foundation for obesity later in life. The sugar added to cow's milk bottle-feeds is sucrose, addictive and fattening, unlike the lactose or milk sugar of breast milk. For the poor, in under-developed countries, the abandonment of breast-feeding is disastrous. In a careful study of children in rural Punjab, published in 1971, Wyon and Gordon concluded: 'In the population studied, virtually all the infants died who did not receive breast-milk in the first months of life.' Even before conception, it is important for the mother and father to be on a good diet which ensures spermatozoa and ova of good quality. And that means a diet rich in protein and fats, especially the essential, unsaturated fats which the body cannot make for itself. An all-meat and fish and poultry diet would be ideal, but a cheaper McCarrison-style version would do equally well (see Chapter 5).

When I was in Toronto in 1959, promoting the first edition of this book, I was taken by a nutritionist friend, Cab Salberston, to see two boys aged about nine and twelve who had recently been shown to a dental convention as examples of perfect teeth and dental arches. They were pleasant, healthy-looking boys and certainly not overweight.

The story their mother told me was that some twelve years earlier just after she had become pregnant with the elder boy, she had heard Stefansson speak at a meeting in Vancouver. So impressed was she with Stefansson's message (that the best food for health was Eskimo-style non-carbohydrate, all-meat with its fat) that she there and then put herself on it and vowed to bring her children up on it. What part her husband played in this I did not discover. Although she was not well off, she stuck to it and by the time I met her, it had become her way of life, and that of her sons. She said it was sometimes difficult for the boys to refuse offers of cookies and sweets from their friends and their parents, but they obeyed their mother and the result was as perfect a pair of physical specimens as I have ever met. I was given the opportunity to question and examine them and I came away convinced that an all-meat, no-carbohydrate diet was right for bringing up children and was particularly good for teeth. Theirs were perfect . . . not a hole or a filling in sight.

This confirmed for me the rightness of what Donaldson said about teeth and their relation to the health of the rest of the body. Later, when he talked to me in London in 1962, he said : 'Cells of which we are made have common nutritional needs. The same food that keeps teeth healthy may prevent cataracts developing in the eyes and may also be good for the cells involved in mysterious diseases like duodenal ulcer, migraine, high blood pressure and obesity.'

So, as part of the summing up in this chapter it can be stated that sound, whole-food nutrition in foetal life, infancy, and childhood, will not only prevent the onset of obesity but will bring the benefits of good health and proper functioning to every cell in the body, including those of the nervous system and the gonads, which are responsible for making those vital cells which will hand life on. The men and women who take heroin, barbiturates and other drugs of addiction such as tobacco, are known to produce substandard sperms and ova which start their offspring off under a handicap. Faulty nutrition in parents will have the same adverse effect. If they do not eat the right building blocks for functionally and structurally healthy cells, the effect on the start they give their children will be as bad as if they were poisoning themselves with drugs.

No discussion of the foundations of obesity in infancy would be complete without mention of the careful work of Dr Jean Mayer, Associate Professor of Nutrition at the Harvard School of Public Health, Boston, Massachusetts. In a talk called 'Genetic Factors in Obesity' (1965), he said:

It is rather amusing that, while misinformed public health educators have denied the importance of genes in the determination of obesity, farmers have recognized and utilized this genetic determination for thousands of years. When animal fat is desired, certain strains predisposed to adiposity are selected in preference to other strains.

Suggestive of the importance of genetic factors in the etiology of human obesity is the finding that segregation can be shown to take place in the transmission of obesity. If the various types of matings, stout × stout, stout × non-stout, and non-stout × non-stout are considered, the variability of weight of the offspring is relatively small for the first type (most [73 per cent in his study] offspring stout), least for the third type (almost none [9 per cent in his study] of the offspring stout), and largest for the stout by non-stout matings (offspring almost evenly divided between obese [41 per cent] and non-obese [59 per cent]). This is interpreted by Gurney as showing that stout individuals carry gametes for slenderness while slender individuals rarely carry gametes for stoutness.

Finally, perhaps the most striking indication of genetic determination in human obesity is the demonstration by Angel that the sex ratios of children in the various types of matings (as characterized by weight) are statistically different from that for the population as a whole.

It is my hope that the evidence presented in this lecture has illustrated a number of points. First, that genetic factors do influence body weight and may cause obesity. Second, that obesity is the common end-product of a great many conditions which may have very little in common except the occurrence of a positive energy balance. Third, that if these conditions differ in mechanism, their treatment ought to differ – for example, if inactivity is an essential aspect of a particular syndrome, increased activity may be more effective than calorie restriction alone. From the point of view of public health, it would appear more profitable to recognize the role of genetic factors and use them to anticipate obesity than to deny obvious facts. The use of genetics has been highly successful in terms of detection and early prevention as regards diabetes. Once it is recognized that the children of obese subjects are much more likely to become obese, preventive efforts could be similarly concentrated on such vulnerable individuals. Proper food and exercise habits could be taught early. All workers in the field are in agreement that the longer obesity has lasted, the more malignant it is apt to be. Recognition of genetic factors may thus help to prevent obesity from ever appearing or at least from developing in many individuals. Once again, our treatment of obesity is likely to be more successful if we view this condition as a medical, rather than a moral, problem.

Genetic Counselling clinics already exist in some areas of Britain, under the NHS. There is one in Southampton serving the Wessex Region (Hampshire, Dorset, Wiltshire and the Isle of Wight). It gives advice mainly on the likelihood of the emergence of serious congenital abnormalities like mongolism and haemophilia, but there is no reason why, in the future, advice about congenital obesity should not be given and appropriate evasive action taken by the prospective parents.

As Jean Mayer says, 'recognition of genetic factors may help to prevent obesity ever appearing', and anyone who has seen a fat child enduring the miseries of teasing and ostracism at school would say 'Amen' to that.

From what I have said so far, it must be obvious that the problem of obesity is not only far more complicated than the calorie-counting pundits would have us believe, but that it is not a single entity. There are many reasons why a person gets too fat, ranging from having the wrong sort of parents, through wrong feeding in the womb and in infancy, through gluttony and food addiction, to hormonal diseases, metabolic disorders and psychological upsets. But I am convinced that the main and commonest cause of obesity is the one we can most easily do something to correct: abuse of the body by giving it the wrong sort of food – refined starches and sugars instead of good, whole food, well grown, particularly meat, fish and poultry *with the fat included*.

In Chapter 1, I told how this sensible and effective treatment for obesity first came to be tried out in the middle of the nineteenth century by Mr Harvey on his patient, William Banting, and went on to give the scientific confirmation of the rightness of this approach by modern medical research workers, notably Professor Kekwick and Dr Pawan at the Middlesex Hospital in London.

In Chapter 2, I exposed the carorie fallacy, and by describing man's evolution in relation to his food, showed that he is an omnivor, best adapted to fat and protein. Just as man's basic mental drives which determine much of his behaviour have not changed in millions of years (see Desmond Morris's two books, *The Naked Ape* and *The Human Zoo*), so his physical adaptation to his food has remained unchanged and there is ample evidence to show that he can avoid obesity and keep his nervous system intact by sticking to the food which helped to determine the change from ape to intelligent man: fat meat.

In Chapter 3, I gave the clinical evidence from doctors all over the world who have shown in their treatment of fat patients – and sometimes their own obesity – that a non-carbohydrate, Stone-Age diet of protein and fat, with no restriction of the amount eaten, will cure obesity every time it is applied.

In Chapter 4, I answered some of the objections often raised against high-fat diets and showed how baseless they are. I also gave an alternative, cheaper dietary approach to overweight which should please vegetarians and others opposed to the eating of meat. It is based on the work of the nutritionist pioneer, Sir Robert McCarrison, and that of Surgeon Captain Cleave who has done more research than anyone else on the high-fibre diet. Being an omnivor, man carries within his cells the enzymatic equipment to deal with unrefined starches and sugars as well as fats and proteins. Trouble comes only when the sugars and starches are concentrated so that they are consumed in quantities far exceeding those taken under the natural conditions in which we evolved.

In Chapter 5, I have given some menus and diet sheets with instructions on how to follow either the Eat-Fat-Grow-Slim diet or the McCarrison/Cleave type of diet based on unprocessed, whole-food cereal grains, fruits, vegetables and dairy products, all raised organically on good soil without chemical additives of any kind.

Chapter 6 deals with some psychiatric aspects of obesity and describes its opposite, that interesting condition *anorexia nervosa*, in which, instead of eating too much or wrongly and becoming fat, the patient seems determined to starve to death – and sometimes does.

Chapter 7 gives details of other ways of slimming, including surgery and drugs. Fasting is dealt with and some recent research mentioned.

In this last chapter, I am attempting to draw all the threads together and give a balanced view of nutrition and obesity, based on over twenty years' study of the subject, first as a general practitioner and now, for the past ten years, as a psychiatrist with a strong leaning towards physical medicine and the somato-psychic approach to mental illness rather than the still dominant psycho-somatic one. (See my new book *Not All in the Mind* (Pan Books) for a development of this theme.)

I have been fortunate for most of my medical life to have had jobs which keep me seeing patients, so that any approach I may use in either psychological or physical medicine has always been tested in practice, not on white mice and rabbits on the laboratory bench but on living men, women and children. These patients have taught me most of what I know and have convinced me that in spite of our much-vaunted scientific knowledge, National Health Service and free education, our health is going downhill at an accelerating pace.

It is true that our children have never looked bonnier, though too many are overweight, or have ever before so easily and successfully escaped or survived the epidemic infections of a century ago which killed off so many in infancy – our churchyards bear witness to this with their hundreds of pathetic little gravestones marking where these children lie. But this is misleading as the pattern of ill-health has changed altogether in the past fifty or sixty years. Until then devastating infections with bacteria and viruses – TB, pneumonia, measles, diphtheria, smallpox, cholera and poliomyelitis, struck down children and people in the prime of life. But we now have a state of affairs in Western affluent societies where degenerative diseases of the heart, arteries and nervous system are putting a load on the health services almost too great for them to bear. And nobody in authority seems to know why.

To me and to colleagues who think like me, the reason is clear: it is due to what we are allowing the food industry to do to our food and drink. With hardly a squeak of protest, we have allowed the vast experiment of altering our nutrition from natural to manufactured foods to be conducted for commercial gain by the giant food-manufacturing combines. Since about 1900 they have been allowed to modify our food in ways which make it totally different from the food on which we evolved so successfully over millions of years.

(1) Wheat and other cereal grains have been robbed of the nutritious germ and necessary fibrous outer layers, which are fed to farm animals, while the human population is sold refined white flour composed almost exclusively of fattening starch with a few additions such as iron, calcium and Vitamin B, which the millers put back so as to be able to claim that the flour they have deliberately impoverished has been 'enriched'.

(2) The consumption of refined white sugar has now reached the staggering figure of 112 lb. per head per annum in Western countries (in Britain the figure is even higher and we have the worst teeth in the world).

(3) Meat has not only become too expensive for most families to eat as much of it as they should, but fish and poultry are going the same way and will soon become luxuries for all but the wealthy, unless this trend is reversed by resolute Government action.

Apart from this phenomenal rise in price, the methods by which livestock for human consumption is reared have changed drastically, and in the intensive farming methods now employed we are seeing a concentration on the production of obesity fat in the animals rather than the vital structural unsaturated fats which free-range animals make and which are essential for the growth and maintenance of a healthy nervous system in the humans who eat them.

(4) Hundreds of new, synthetic chemicals are being added to food at every stage in its production: colourings, flavours, sweeteners, anti-oxidants, preservatives, bleachers, antibiotics, all to make the food look, smell or taste better, and to last longer without going bad. And the motive? Profit, and the need to feed more people than the planet can comfortably support.

To the people who say we have never been so fit or better fed, I answer that inability to measure damage to health does *not* mean that damage does not exist. And the stark evidence of our degenerative deterioration in the West is there for all to read in the appalling, rising number of deaths from strokes and coronary thrombosis. Dr Paul Dudley White, President Eisenhower's physician at the time of his heart attacks, saw his first case in 1920. Today 500,000 die annually of heart attacks in the USA, 70–80,000 in Britain. Atherosclerosis – the forerunner of heart attacks and strokes – is confined to people taking the altered diet I have described above. A small number of people in Western countries, aware of the dangers, have put themselves on a Stone-Age or McCarrison-type diet. They constitute a most important group for investigation and should be sought out and put into a prospective study without delay, matched with a group taking the ordinary, Western, supermarket diet.

From a short monograph on obesity, published in 1958, this book has evolved into a study of our Western way of eating. And as a spin-off has enabled me to take a new look at psychiatry in relation to diet and to show that many chronic mental patients can be rehabilitated without drugs, electric shocks or operations on the brain, simply by eliminating certain new, chemically-adulterated foods from their diets. The mind and body are one and the mind is really the manifestation of the physical brain in action. If wrong food can make people fat and rot their teeth, why should it not, in some susceptible people, injure their brains as well and make them appear mad?

References to Chapter 8

p. 180 'The Baby Killer', published by War on Want, 467 Caledonian Road, London N7 9BE.

p. 180 *Present-Day Practice in Infant Feeding*, Department of Health, HMSO.

p. 181 Fattening effect of adding sucrose to bottle feeds:
Nutritional Review, 1973, *31*, p. 116.
Jelliffe, D. B., *British Medical Journal*, 1973, *2*, p. 546.

p. 181 Fatal effects on infants in the Punjab of failure to breast feed:
Wyon, J. B., and Gordon, J. E., *The Khanna Study*, Harvard, 1971, p. 187.

p. 182 Genetic factors in obesity:
Angel, J. L., 'Constitution in Female Obesity', *American Journal of Physical Anthropology*, 1949, 7, pp. 433–471.
Gurney, R., *Archives of Internal Medicine*, 1936, 57, pp. 557–561.
Mayer, J., *Annals of New York Academy of Science*, 1965, vol. 131, p. 412.

APPENDIX A

Tables of Normal Weight for Height and Build (Based on Life Insurance Tables)

These heights and weights are approximations only, based on statistical information. The division into three columns according to body type has been made in order to help people wanting to slim to choose a realistic target weight for themselves. Decide first to which of the three basic body types you belong and then work to that column of weights. Base your judgement on your shape before you became so fat that you wanted to slim.

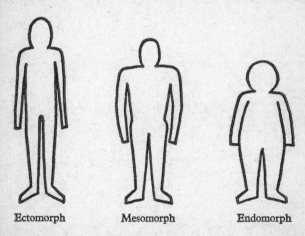

Ectomorph   Mesomorph   Endomorph

Ectomorphs are basically tall, thin people with poorly developed muscles, long backs and slender hands and feet. They do not usually become obese and are the prototype Constant-Weights. Frequently they are underweight.

Mesomorphs have wide shoulders and narrow hips with powerful muscles. They tend to be good at athletics and when they stop taking regular, vigorous exercise, tend to put on excess fat.

Endomorphs are usually short in stature, have large body cavities (chest and abdomen) and short arms and legs with pudgy hands and small feet. They are the Fatten-Easilies.

It is unrealistic for a fat person who comes from a long line of endomorphs to imagine that by dieting he will turn himself into an ectomorph. But he *can* get down to his proper weight for his height and build. Similarly, ectomorphs who are too thin and light, can get up to their normal weight on the Eat-Fat-Grow-Slim regime. (See Chapter 3 for the story of Dr Lutz.)

NORMAL WEIGHTS FOR MEN OF AGES 25 AND OVER

Weight in pounds according to build (in ordinary clothes)

Height (without shoes)		ecto-morph	meso-morph	endo-morph
Feet	Inches			
5	2	116-125	124-133	131-142
5	3	119-128	127-136	133-144
5	4	122-132	130-140	137-149
5	5	126-136	134-144	141-153
5	6	129-139	137-147	145-157
5	7	133-143	141-151	149-162
5	8	136-147	145-156	153-166
5	9	140-151	149-160	157-170
5	10	144-155	153-164	161-175
5	11	148-159	157-168	165-180
6	0	152-164	161-173	169-185
6	1	157-169	166-178	174-190
6	2	163-175	171-184	179-196
6	3	168-180	176-189	184-202

NORMAL WEIGHT FOR WOMEN OF AGES 25 AND OVER

Weight in pounds according to build (in ordinary clothes)

Height (without shoes) Feet	Inches	ecto	meso	endo
4	11	104-111	110-118	117-127
5	0	105-113	112-120	119-129
5	1	107-115	114-122	121-131
5	2	110-118	117-125	124-135
5	3	113-121	120-128	127-138
5	4	116-125	124-132	131-142
5	5	119-128	127-135	133-145
5	6	123-132	130-140	138-150
5	7	126-136	134-144	142-154
5	8	129-139	137-147	145-158
5	9	133-143	141-151	149-162
5	10	136-147	145-155	152-166
5	11	139-150	148-158	155-169

Quick-Reference Table to Non-Carbohydrate Foods

Based on the data in the M.R.C. revised (1964) edition of
Chemical Composition of Foods by McCance
and Widdowson

You may eat as much as you like of these

*** very high fat.
** more fat than protein.
* fat and protein about equal.
unstarred items have more protein than fat

MEAT, POULTRY AND GAME

	Protein: Fat Ratio			Protein: Fat Ratio	
Bacon, raw Danish, Wilts, average	4.0:	10.6**	Beefsteak stewed	8.7:	2.4
Ditto fore end	4.2:	9.0**	Brain, boiled	3.4:	1.6
Ditto middle	3.7:	12.7**	Chicken, boiled	7.4:	2.9
Ditto gammon	4.3:	8.0**	Chicken, roast	8.4:	2.1
Beef, corned	6.3:	4.3	Dripping, beef	tr.:	28.1***
Beef, silverside boiled	7.9:	5.7*	Duck, roast	6.5:	6.7
Beef, sirloin, lean and fat	6.0:	9.1**	Goose, roast	8.0:	6.4
Beef steak, fried	5.8:	5.8*	Grouse, roast	8.6:	1.5
Beef steak, grilled	7.2:	6.1*	Ham, boiled, lean and fat	4.6:	11.2**
Liver, fried	8.3:	4.1	Heart, roast	7.1:	4.2
Mutton chop, grilled, lean and fat	4.4:	17.1***	Kidney, stewed	7.3:	1.6
			Kidney, fried	7.9:	2.6
			Pork leg, roast	7.0:	6.6*
			Pork loin, roast, lean and fat	6.7:	4.5
Mutton leg, boiled	7.3:	4.7	Pork chops, grilled	5.3:	14.3***
			Rabbit, stewed	7.6:	2.2

Protein: Fat Ratio

Mutton leg, roast	7.1:	5.8*	Tongue	5.4:	6.8**
			Tripe, stewed	5.1:	0.9
Mutton scrag and neck, stewed	5.2:	5.2*	Turkey, roast	8.6:	2.2
			Veal cutlet, fried	8.6:	2.3
Pheasant, roast	5.5:	1.7	Venison, roast	9.5:	1.8

****Normal serving will balance an* x *on the fruit and vegetable list.*

***Larger serving will balance an* x *on the fruit and vegetable list.*

x *against fruits or vegetables means they contain enough carbohydrate to stop you losing weight if you eat a lot of them.*

FISH

Protein: Fat Ratio

Bloaters, grilled	6.4:	4.9*	Haddock, fried	5.8:	2.4
Bream, steamed	3.3:	0.6	Haddock, smoked steamed	6.3:	0.3
Cockles	3.1:	0.1			
Cod, steamed	5.1:	0.3	Hake, steamed	5.2:	0.9
Cod, fried	5.9:	1.3	Hake, fried	5.5:	3.2
Cod, grilled	7.7:	1.5	Halibut, steamed	6.4:	1.1
Cod roe, fried	5.8:	3.4			
Crab, boiled	5.4:	1.5	Herring, fried	6.2:	4.3*
Eels, stewed	5.0:	9.2*	Herring, baked in vinegar	4.8:	3.7*
Flounder, fried	4.8:	3.7*			
Haddock, steamed	6.2:	0.2	Herring roe, fried	6.6:	4.5*
Kippers	6.6:	3.2	Scallops, steamed	6.4:	0.4
Lobster, boiled	6.0:	1.0			
Mackerel, fried	5.7:	3.2	Shrimps	6.3:	0.7
Mussels, raw	3.3:	0.5	Skate, fried	4.3:	4.7*
Mussels, boiled	4.8:	0.6	Sole, steamed	5.0:	0.4
Oysters, raw	2.9:	0.3	Sole, fried	5.7:	5.2*
Pilchards, tinned	6.2:	3.1	Sprats, fried	6.3:	10.8*
			Trout, steamed	6.3:	1.3
Plaice, steamed	5.1:	0.5	Turbot, steamed	5.9:	0.5
Plaice, fried	5.1:	4.1	Whitebait, fried	5.2:	13.5**

Protein: Fat Ratio			*Protein: Fat Ratio*		
Prawns	6.0:	0.5	Whiting,		
Salmon, fresh			steamed	5.7:	0.3
steamed	5.4:	3.7	Whiting, fried	4.4:	2.6
Sardines, tinned	5.8:	6.4*	Winkles boiled in		
			salt water	4.3:	0.4

DAIRY PRODUCTS

Protein: Fat Ratio			*Protein: Fat Ratio*		
Butter, fresh	0.1:	24.2***	Egg yolk	4.6:	8.7*
Cheese,			Eggs,		
cheddar	7.1:	9.8**	raw/boiled	3.4:	3.5*
Cheese, cream	0.9:	24.5***	Eggs, dried	12.3:	12.3*
Cheese, Dutch	8.0:	4.8	Eggs, fried	4.0:	5.5**
Cheese, gorgon-			Eggs, poached	3.5:	3.3*
zola	7.1:	8.8*	¶Milk, fresh		
Cheese,			whole	0.9:	1.1*
Gruyère	10.4:	9.5*	¶Milk, fresh		
Cheese, packet	6.4:	5.4*	skimmed	1.0:	0.1
Cheese,			¶Milk, condensed		
parmesan	9.8:	8.4*	whole unsweet-		
Cheese, St Ivel	6.6:	8.7**	ened	2.2:	2.4
Cheese, Stilton	7.1:	11.4**	¶Milk, dried		
Cream	0.5:	11.9***	skimmed house-		
Egg white	2.6:	0	hold	9.7:	0.1

¶*These contain carbohydrate and must not be taken freely—limit half-pint a day.*

REFERENCE TABLE TO LOW-CARBOHYDRATE FOODS

Some of these must be restricted as indicated.

> x *Stop, only one helping a day*
> o *Caution*
> † *Go, eat as much as you like*

VEGETABLES

	Protein:	Carbohydrate		Protein:	Carbohydrate
Asparagus	1.0:	0.3 †	Leeks	0.5:	1.3 o
Beans, broad			Lettuce	0.3:	0.5 †
boiled	1.2:	2.0 o	Marrow	0.1:	0.4 †
Beans, french	0.2:	0.3 †	Mushrooms	0.5:	0.0 †
Beans, haricot	1.9:	4.7 x	Onions	0.2:	0.8 †
Beans, runner	0.2:	0.3 †	Parsnips	0.4:	3.8 x
Beetroot	0.5:	2.8 x	Peas	1.4:	2.2 o
Brussels sprouts	0.7:	0.5 †	Potatoes, boiled	0.4:	5.6 x
Cabbage	0.4:	0.3 †	Pumpkin	0.6:	3.4 x
Carrots	0.3:	1.3 o	Radishes	0.3:	0.8 †
Cauliflower	0.4:	0.3 †	Spinach	1.4:	0.4 †
Celery, raw	0.3:	0.4 †	Spring Greens	0.5:	0.3 †
Celery, boiled	0.2:	0.2 †	Swedes	0.3:	1.1 o
Chicory	0.2:	0.4 †	Tomatoes, raw	0.3:	0.8 †
Cucumber	0.2:	0.5 †	Turnips	0.4:	0.7 †
			Watercress	0.2:	0.2 †

† *are low carbohydrate and may be taken freely.*
o *are medium carbohydrate and should be taken only in moderation.*
x *are relatively high carbohydrate and should be restricted to one*
  serving a day and balanced with one of the high fat (***) or
  (**) foods in the Meat, Fish and Dairy Products lists.

FRUITS

Stewed fruit must not be sweetened with sugar
Tinned fruit should be avoided unless known to be sugar-free.

Protein: Carbohydrate				*Protein: Carbohydrate*		
Apples, eating	0.1:	3.3	o	Greengages,		
Apples, baked	0.1:	2.3	o	stewed	0.1:	2.2 o
Apples, stewed	—:	1.2	o	Lemon juice	0.1:	0.5 †
Apricots	0.2:	1.7	o	Loganberries	0.2:	1.0 †
Apricots, dried				Melons,		
stewed	0.6:	5.1	x	cantaloupe	0.3:	1.5 o
Bananas	0.2:	5.5	x	Oranges	0.2:	1.8 o
Blackberries, raw	0.4:	1.8	o	Orange juice	0.2:	2.7 o
Blackberries,				Peaches	0.2:	2.3 o
stewed	0.2:	0.9	o	Pears	0.1:	3.0 o
Cherries	0.1:	3.0	o	Pears, stewed	0.1:	1.8 o
Damsons	0.1:	1.8	o	Pineapple	0.1:	3.3 o
Damsons,				Plums	0.2:	2.7 o
stewed	0.1:	1.8	o	Plums, stewed	0.1:	1.1 o
Figs	0.4:	2.7	o	Prunes, stewed	0.3:	4.4 o
Gooseberries,				Rasberries,		
stewed	0.2:	0.5	†	stewed	0.2:	1.1 o
Grapes, black	0.2:	4.4	o	Rhubarb, stewed	0.1:	0.2 †
Grapes, white	0.2:	4.6	o	Strawberries	0.2:	1.8 o
Grapefruit	0.1:	0.7	†			

† *are low carbohydrate and may be taken freely.*
o *are medium carbohydrate and should be taken only in moderation.*
x *are relatively high carbohydrate and should be restricted to one*
   serving a day and balanced with one of the high fat (***) or
   (**) foods in the Meat, Fish and Dairy Products lists.

Appendix B

NUTS

	Protein	:	Fat	Carbohydrate
Almonds	5.8	:	15.2	1.2 0
Barcelona	3.7	:	18.2	1.5 0
Brazil	3.9	:	17.3	1.2 0
Chestnuts	0.7	:	0.8	10.4 x
Cob nuts	2.6	:	10.2	1.9 0
Coconut, fresh	1.1	:	10.2	1.1 0
Coconut, desiccated	1.9	:	17.2	1.8 0
Peanuts	8.0	:	13.9	2.4 0
Walnuts	3.6	:	14.6	1.4 0
Olives (with stone)	0.2	:	2.5	negligible

APPENDIX C

Menus For a Week at a Glance

These are suggestions for people who may run short of ideas for Eat-Fat-Grow-Slim meals.

All the items are interchangeable and by picking out the less expensive ones and repeating them, the cost may be reduced.

MONDAY

Breakfast
½ grapefruit and saccharine or saxin (no sugar)
Coffee and top milk, no sugar
Two rashers bacon and egg

Lunch
Tomato juice (unsweetened)
Veal steak with gravy made from fat it was fried in (no flour) or
Corned beef
With boiled french beans
Cheese soufflé or Cheddar cheese

Tea
Tea with lemon
Pot of yoghourt

Supper
Clear vegetable soup made with meat stock
Tinned salmon
Green salad and tomatoes, oil and vinegar
Cream cheese
A cup of milk

TUESDAY

Breakfast
Tomato juice (unsweetened)
Haddock (large portion) stewed in milk with 2 pats butter
Coffee with cream or top milk

Lunch
½ grapefruit
Cod's roes on salad (or sardines in oil on salad)
Fresh fruit salad unsweetened and fresh cream
Coffee and cream

Tea
Tea with lemon
Fresh fruit salad unsweetened and cream

Supper
Beef steak
Fried tomatoes
Watercress
Cheese

WEDNESDAY

Breakfast

Fresh orange juice
Fresh ham with fat
Fried egg
Coffee with cream or top milk

Lunch

Cold buttered prawns, *or*
Jellied eels
Green salad with mayonnaise
  made with cream
Black coffee and cream
Wedge of Gruyère cheese

Tea

Tea with lemon (no sugar)
Fresh fruit salad and cream

Supper

Glass of grapefruit juice
Large portion of beef stew
  with vegetables, no potatoes
Black coffee with cream

THURSDAY

Breakfast

Fresh orange juice
Fried kidneys
Fried tomatoes
Coffee and cream or top milk

Lunch

Tomato juice
Corned beef
Peas (¾ cup)
Brie or Cheddar cheese

Tea

Tea with lemon
Fresh fruit salad unsweetened
  and cream

Supper

Asparagus soup (no thickening)
Lamb, mint sauce
½ cup broad beans with butter
Plums and unsweetened cream

FRIDAY

Breakfast

½ grapefruit
Omelette
Coffee and cream or top milk

Lunch

2 slices of melon
Tuna fish (tinned) or whelks
  or winkles
Peas (¾ cup)
Rhubarb unsweetened and
  cream

Tea

Tea with lemon
Yoghourt

Supper

Mussels or ½ avocado pear and
  salad dressing
Liver and bacon, fried
Creamed spinach (2 cups)
Coffee and cream

SATURDAY	SUNDAY

Breakfast

Fresh orange juice
Bran flakes and cream
Fried eggs
Coffee with cream or top milk

Breakfast

Tomato juice
Coffee with cream or top milk
Eggs (scrambled with butter)

Lunch

½ grapefruit
Steak and salad
Cheddar cheese
Black coffee and cream

Lunch

Roast beef and cabbage, small portion chips or boiled potato
Fresh fruit salad unsweetened and cream
Black coffee and cream

Tea

Tea with lemon
2 glasses buttermilk

Supper

Sweetbreads with broad beans (2 oz.)
Fresh pineapple and cream
Black coffee

Supper

Tripe and onions
Cheese and salad
Large coffee and cream

REMEMBER: No sugar, no bread, no flour for thickening, not much added salt. Saccharine or Saxin may be used for sweetening and there is no restriction on water. Drink at least 3 pints a day, flavoured with fresh lemon juice if you like it.

The Grant Loaf

(Adapted for sugar-free diet)

Quantities for two loaves:

- 2 lb. wholewheat, stone-ground flour (7 American standard cup measures)
- 26 fluid oz. (a generous pint) of water at blood heat (3 American standard cup measures)
- 1 heaped teaspoon of salt, or according to taste
- 2 level British standard teaspoons of dried yeast (DCL brand, tinned, works well)

Method:

Mix the salt with the flour (in very cold weather, warm the flour slightly, enough to take off the chill). Place in a cup 2 tablespoons of water at blood heat; the temperature is important, so check with a cooking thermometer which should read 35° to 38° Centigrade. Sprinkle the dried yeast on top of the water. In about 15 minutes this should have produced a creamy froth. Pour this into the flour and add the rest of the water. Mix well by hand for a minute or so, working from the sides to the middle, until the dough feels elastic and does not stick to the sides of the mixing bowl. Divide the dough, which should be slippery but not wet, into two two-pint tins which have been warmed and well-greased. Put the tins in a warm place, cover with a cloth and leave for 20 minutes or until the dough has risen to within half an inch of the tops of the tins. Bake in a fairly hot oven: electricity 400° F., gas Regulo 6, for 35 to 40 minutes.

The Bran-Plus Loaf

(Adapted for sugar-free diet)

Using same method as for Grant Loaf, above

Quantities for two loaves:

- 2 lb. wholewheat, stone-ground flour (7 American standard cups)

3 oz. fresh, unprocessed bran (1 scant American standard cup)
1 heaped teaspoon of salt, or according to taste
2 level British standard teaspoons of dried yeast
28 fluid oz. of water at blood heat – just under 1½ pints (3½
   American standard cup measures)

This Bran-Plus loaf has a delicious, nutty flavour. The special
water-holding properties of the bran keeps it moist and new-
tasting even when 3 or 4 days old. If properly made it can be
cut easily into thin slices, even when new. It is particularly
recommended for people with constipation or irritable colon.

HINTS

The flour. This should be stone-ground and, ideally, should
be made from wheat which has been organically grown. Most
health shops stock it and also some supermarkets, but the
demand is now becoming greater than the supply. Farmers
might be induced to grow wheat this way, however, if they
could sell it at more than the guaranteed price.

The water. The simplest way of obtaining water at blood heat
without a thermometer is by putting half a pint of boiling water
in a 2-pint measure jug and filling it up with stone-cold water.
(Blood heat is approximately 35–38° Centigrade or 95–100°
Fahrenheit.) The quantity of water varies slightly with the type
of flour. Some flours need a little more than 2 pints, some need
less. The right consistency of the dough is soon found after very
little experience.

The salt. This should be table sea-salt or Malvern salt. Be
sparing with salt as too much prevents the yeast from raising
the dough sufficiently.

The yeast. If ordinary baker's yeast is used, it will keep very
well, refrigerated, for four or five days, if placed in a plastic
bag, *inside its own paper bag.* If dried yeast is used, and this is
more convenient, follow the directions carefully and *be sure to
close the tin firmly after use.* If the dough is allowed to rise too
high, dried yeast can impart a yeasty taste to the bread which
some people find unpleasant.

Rising the dough. If there is difficulty in finding a warm place in which to place the tins while the dough is rising, put them covered with a cloth on the rack over your gas or electric cooker and turn one of the hot-plates to very low.

The Whole Food Diet for Weight Reduction and Good Health

(Reprinted by permission of *Harpers and Queen* magazine)

On Waking

The juice of a lemon in a glass of warm water.

Breakfast

A bowl of yoghourt sprinkled with a teaspoon of wheatgerm and a tablespoon of bran.

Fresh fruit: an apple, pear, melon, bunch of grapes, slice of fresh pineapple.

Decaffeinated coffee with skim milk if desired.

Lunch

A glass of fresh fruit or vegetable juice.

A large raw salad. Choose three or more of these foods and mix together: lettuce, chicory, watercress, beet tops, chopped apple, white heart of cabbage, carrots, radishes, raw sliced mushrooms, red and green peppers, spring onions, cucumbers.

Then add: 2 to 4 ounces of milled sunflower seeds and mixed nuts (can be milled in a coffee grinder or blender), 2 to 4 ounces of curd, or cottage cheese (or have a wedge of Camembert on the side).

Dressing: one tablespoon of safflower or sunflower oil mixed with 1 teaspoon apple cider vinegar or lemon juice. (You can add herbs, fresh garlic, and pepper for flavour.)

Sweet: Live yoghourt with a teaspoon of frozen orange juice concentrate for sweetening (no sugar, please); or fresh fruit salad.

Decaffeinated coffee, or tea with a slice of lemon.

Dinner

A glass of fresh fruit or vegetable juice or a serving of melon. 4 ounces of grilled or braised lean meat; or 6 ounces of baked or grilled or steamed fish; or an unfired nut rissole (see recipe, p. 209). A cooked vegetable if desired (broccoli, brussels sprouts, asparagus, courgettes, etc.) with a dab of butter or Flora.

A mixed green salad (condiments as at lunch).

Sweet: as at lunch.
Decaffeinated coffee, Pioneer or herb tea.

If you work in an office, before you leave in the morning fill a plastic bag with raw carrots, celery, green peppers and raw mushrooms to take with you . . . at home keep a bowl of them at hand in the fridge for 'nibblers' any time. You may also have Potassium Broth, herb tea, or decaffeinated coffee and up to 4 ounces of sunflower seeds a day between meals. If you have no weight problem, add to this diet three slices of whole grain bread per day, and sweets made with wholegrain flours, raw sugar, honey, or dried fruit. *Eliminate completely white sugar, all refined flours and products containing them and all pre-cooked, packaged, processed foods.* Check with your doctor before beginning this regime.

Recipes

High energy drink (if you want a booster for a hard day)

Juice of two fresh oranges;
Same amount of water;
1 raw egg;
1 teaspoon of brewer's yeast powder;
1 dessertspoon of wheatgerm
1 tablespoon of honey;
1 dessertspoon of skim milk powder.

Blend well and serve.

Unfired nut rissoles

4 oz. of milled sunflower seeds (can be made in a coffee grinder
      or blender);
4 oz. of milled mixed nuts (brazils, cashews, hazels, almonds);
1 tablespoon of soya flour;
4 oz. of grated raw carrot with a little lemon juice.

Mix ingredients together with 4 tablespoons of live yoghourt or
two raw eggs, add soy sauce, or chopped chives, and a few
herbs or a little crushed garlic if desired. Make into small patties
to be stored in the refrigerator . . . they will keep for five days
and 'travel' well for taking to work for lunch, etc.

Potassium Broth

(Excellent for that 'nervy' feeling when you are slimming and
to stop any tendency to muscle cramps.)

Using a stainless steel, enamel, or earthenware pot, fill it with
two pints of water then slice vegetables directly into it (to
prevent oxidation). Use at least 4 stalks of celery (root and leaf
included); 1 cup of diced or shredded carrots; a bulb of fennel
with leaves chopped; turnip tops, parsley, or beet tops as available; a few spring onions. Add several leaves of lemon thyme
and a bay leaf. Cover and cook slowly for 45 minutes at least.
Let stand until cool. Strain, and serve hot or cold with a pinch
of Herbamare.

The broth can be refrigerated for two or three days until needed.
It can be drunk at any time of the day and is a good between-
meal vitalizer. (You can vary the formula with other vegetables
as they are in season.)

Glossary of Medical Terms

ADIPOSE Fat, fatty.

AMINO-ACIDS Basic components of proteins. There are many. All contain the amino (NH_2) group and the carboxyl (COOH) group.

AMPHETAMINES Known also under proprietary names, 'Benzedrine' and 'Dexedrine'. Chemicals related to ephedrine and having the power to shrink swollen mucous membranes after local application and to cause wakefulness and depress appetite.

ATHEROMA From the Greek words meaning porridge tumour. Fatty plaques which appear on the inner lining of arteries in degenerative arterial disease, e.g. arteriosclerosis.

BIOCHEMISTRY The chemistry of living organisms and vital processes.

CALORIE A unit of heat. The amount of heat required to raise 1 kilogram of water from 15° C. to 16° C.

CAPSULE From the Latin word meaning a little box. The capsule of a joint is a membranous envelope enclosing the fluid which acts as a lubricant, facilitating movement.

CARBOHYDRATE So named because the hydrogen and oxygen are usually present in the same proportion as in water, combined with carbon. They include the starches, sugars, celluloses and gums.

CATALYTIC From the Greek word meaning to dissolve or break down. A catalyst changes the velocity of a chemical reaction without itself entering into the reaction. Its mere presence has the effect.

CHOLESTEROL From the Greek words meaning bile solids. A fat-like, pearly substance, it is a common constituent of gall-stones. Cholesterol is found all over the healthy body and in atheroma and cancer tissue. It is vital to life.

DIABETIC From the Greek words meaning a syphon, or to go through. Diabetes is a disease marked by the discharge of an excessive quantity of urine.

Diabetes mellitus (sugar-diabetes in popular speech) is the type of diabetes usually referred to. It is a metabolic disorder in which the ability to oxidize carbohydrates is lost to a greater or lesser degree. The cause is a fault in the islets of Langerhans, in the pancreas, which fail to produce enough of the hormone insulin.

Symptoms are thirst, sugar in the urine, which is passed in excessive amounts, hunger, weakness and, in severe cases, coma.

ENZYMES From the Greek words meaning 'in yeast'. An enzyme is an organic chemical, often a protein, capable of transforming one compound into another by catalytic action.

EPIDEMIOLOGY From three Greek words meaning general-among-people. The branch of science which deals with the relationships between the various factors determining the frequency and distribution of disease among population groups.

EXOPTHALMIC From two Greek words meaning 'out' and 'eye'. Abnormal protrusion of the eyeball. Seen most often in thyrotoxicosis, from over-action of the thyroid gland.

GLUCOSE From the Greek word meaning sweet. Known also as dextrose, a simple sugar made by breaking down starch.

Liquid glucose, a syrupy fluid, is called corn syrup in America.

GLYCOGEN From the Greek words meaning to produce sweetness. It is a carbohydrate made in the liver from simpler carbohydrates and used in the body either to break down to sugar for energy or as a stepping stone to the synthesis of fat.

GOITRE An enlargement of the thyroid gland causing a swelling in the front part of the neck.

HAEMORRHAGE From two Greek words meaning 'blood' and 'burst forth'. An escape of blood from the veins or arteries. Bleeding.

HERNIA The protrusion of a loop of an organ or tissue through an abnormal opening. The most usual sites are through the navel and in the neighbourhood of the genital organs. Popularly known as 'rupture'.

HORMONE From the Greek word meaning to 'excite' or 'arouse'. A chemical substance produced in a ductless gland which, when transported in the blood to some other organ, produces there a stimulant or inhibitory effect.

HYPERTENSION Abnormally high blood pressure.

HYPOTHALAMUS A region of the brain below the thalamus

(seat of emotion), joining it to the pituitary gland below. It contains regulatory centres for many vital functions not normally under control of the will.

INSULIN A protein hormone capable of lowering the blood sugar and turning sugar into fat. Essential for the metabolism of carbohydrate.

Marketed in vials for the treatment of diabetics who cannot make enough insulin themselves.

ISCHAEMIC From the Greek meaning 'holding back blood'. Pertaining to local or temporary deficiency of blood due to narrowing of a blood vessel. Ischaemic heart disease is often associated with atheroma and coronary thrombosis.

ISOTOPES From the Greek words meaning 'equal place'. Two or more chemical elements which are identical except that they differ in atomic weight or in the structure of the nucleus.

KETONES Acidic substances, related to acetone, formed in the body from the incomplete oxidation of fatty acids and certain proteins.

The prefix ket- signifies the presence of a carbonyl group $C:O$.

KETOSIS A condition charac-terized by excessive formation of ketones in the body.

LECITHIN From the Greek word meaning 'yolk of egg'. A fatty substance containing phosphorus and found in many animal tissues – e.g. nerves, blood and bile.

METABOLISM From a Greek word meaning 'change'. The sum of all the chemical and physical processes by which the living body is produced and maintained.

It also means the trans-formation by which heat and energy are made available in the body. The basal metabolism, BMR or basal metabolic rate, means the minimum heat produced by a person 14 to 18 hours after eating, at rest but not sleeping. It represents the energy used to maintain the basic functions of the body – breathing, digestion, muscle tone, hormone pro-duction, etc.

It is usually expressed in calories per hour per square metre of body surface. A more useful way of express-ing it, when studying the obese, is as calories per hour per unit of body weight.

MOLECULE From the Latin meaning 'little mass'. An aggregation of two or more atoms to form a spe-

chemical substance. The number of atoms in any molecule varies with the type of chemical compound.

MYOCARDIAL Pertaining to the heart muscle.

MYXOEDEMA From two Greek words meaning 'muscle' and 'swelling'. A disease due to lack of thyroid in adults characterized by swelling of the face and hands, slow pulse, dry skin and mental dullness.

Administration of thyroid hormone brings improvement.

OEDEMA Swelling, due to the presence of an abnormal amount of fluid in the intercellular spaces of the body.

ORBIT The bony socket in the skull which contains the eye.

OXIDIZE To combine or cause to combine with oxygen.

PEMMICAN A preparation of dried meat and fat used as a food by the North American Indians. It contains no carbohydrate.

PROTEINS Nitrogen-containing compounds, combinations of amino-acids, which form the basis of the tissues of living animals. Widely distributed in nature, they cannot be absorbed into the body whole, but only after breakdown by the digestive juices into their constituent amino-acids.

PROTOPLASM From the Greek meaning 'first mould'. The only known form of matter in which life is manifested. Composed mainly of water, with proteins, lipids, carbohydrates and mineral salts suspended in colloidal solution.

PSYCHOTHERAPY That form of treatment of mental disorders which employs psychological methods, including suggestion, persuasion, psychoanalysis, exhortation, explanation, etc.

RADIOACTIVE Capable of spontaneous decomposition to give off alpha, beta, or gamma rays. Ordinary chemical substances can be made radioactive by bombarding them with high-velocity particles.

SCURVY Vitamin deficiency disease due to lack of Vitamin C (ascorbic acid) in the diet.

SPHINCTER From the Greek meaning 'a binder'. A ring of muscle which closes a natural orifice.

STEATORRHOEA From two Greek words meaning 'a flow of fat'. A disease characterized by an excess of fat in the stools.

SUBCUTANEOUS Under the skin.

TACHYCARDIA From two Greek words meaning 'swift heart'. Usually applied as a clinical term to a pulse rate above 100 per minute.

TRANSFERENCE In psychiatry, means the shifting of emotion from one person to another, especially by the patient to the analyst, of affection or hostility, based on unconscious identification of the analyst with someone from the patient's own life, e.g. father or mother. If the transference is favourable it is called positive; if unfavourable, negative or counter-transference.

UMBILICUS Navel.

VITAMINS Substances, unrelated chemically, occurring in small amounts in various foods and essential for the normal functioning of the body.

Index